I0114051

After 60

After 60

The **secrets**
to achieving
happiness, health,
and **fulfillment**
in **later life**

Part I

AUDREY C. RALPH, R.N.
GORDON RALPH

Ternion Press

Portland, Oregon

After 60
The secrets to achieving happiness, health, and
fulfillment in later life – Part I
Book 1 in the *Life After 60*™ series
Copyright © 2020 by Ternion Press, LLC

All rights reserved.
No part of this publication may be reproduced, stored in a retrieval system
or transmitted in any form or by any means, electronic, mechanical, photo-
copying, recording, scanning, or otherwise, without the prior written per-
mission of the publisher.

Cover design by Teddi Black
Book design by Sue Balcer

ISBN Hard Cover: 978-1-952887-04-8
ISBN paperback: 978-1-952887-01-7
ISBN e-book: 978-1-952887-00-0

Library of Congress Control Number: 2021908108

Published by Ternion Press, LLC
Portland, Oregon
www.ternionpress.com

First Edition

Disclaimer
The authors' opinions expressed herein are based on both their personal observations and their research and readings on the subject matter.
The authors' opinions may not be universally applicable to all people
in all circumstances. The information presented in this book is in no
way intended as medical advice or as a substitute for medical or other
counseling. The publisher and authors disclaim liability for any negative
or other medical outcomes that may occur as a result of acting on or not
acting on anything set forth in this book.

DEDICATION

To my nieces, Gail and Pam,
for always being there to give me a hand in times of need,
and for bringing pleasure and fun into my life.

Audrey C. Ralph

To my wife, Beth,
for always encouraging me to be my best.

Gordon Ralph

ACKNOWLEDGEMENTS

We have always heard that nothing is produced in a vacuum; that it takes the organized effort of several people to produce anything. The same holds true for this book.

The authors wish to thank the many people who contributed to make this book possible: Karin Maday, who served as an early reader, participated in the cover and title selection test group, and provided the feedback and encouragement to keep going; Tanya Mead, for providing early encouragement and for her edits of this book's early drafts; Sheryl Barbin, who served as a reader, took part in the cover and title selection test group, and provided the encouragement and feedback to keep going. Paul Nimey, who served as a reader and provided the encouragement and feedback to keep going; Teddi Black, for her amazing cover design skills; Lee Caleca, for the excellent line and copy editing she provided during the later drafts of this book; Connie Mableson, for providing a literary review and legal guidance with respect to this, and future books in this series; Sue Balcer, for her expert and meticulous typesetting skills.

Without the help and encouragement of these individuals, this book would have never seen the light of day.

TABLE OF CONTENTS

AUTHORS' NOTES

Throughout my life, I have worked with many of my friends and patients during difficult times. I have gained many ideas and techniques which have hopefully helped them on their path to recovery – healing them both emotionally and physically. I hope that, in sharing some of these methods and techniques, I can contribute in some way to helping you lead a happier, healthier, and more fulfilled life. I am eager to hear from you, and hear how your own personal journey is progressing. Please feel free to write me anytime.

Audrey C. Ralph, R.N. (retired) – Fort Washington, Pennsylvania, February 9th 2020 – acralph@ternionpress.com

---

It is February 2020, and my mom turns 90 this month. Last year, as I sat and reflected on her life and career, I realized that she spent the majority of it caring for older adults; helping them to live happier, healthier, and more fulfilled lives. I also remember thinking that it was *a shame* she never shared her secrets with the world. Suddenly, I said to myself, "what's wrong with now?" Thus began the journey of writing this book.

I view my role in this book as something of a journalist. My goal is to take my mom's teachings, and report them in a factual, entertaining, and engaging way. She supplied the methods and techniques, and I tried to capture and present them to the best of my abilities.

It is my hope that you find this book not only helpful, but also entertaining. I am also sincerely grateful to be able to share my mom's discoveries with you, and hope that they work to improve the quality of your life – just as they have done for countless others she has cared for over the years.

Gordon Ralph – Plymouth Meeting, Pennsylvania, February 9th 2020 – garalph@ternionpress.com

CHAPTER 1

⌒⟶

Bob's First Meeting

Bob sits quietly in the therapist's office. *How the hell did I ever find the courage to come here?* he thinks.

Life hadn't always been so easy for Bob. Even though he was the son of well-educated parents, his father hadn't lived up to his potential and died when Bob was just entering his teenage years. His dad died without insurance, leaving his mom and him nearly destitute. Initially a poor student, Bob learned how to become an excellent student and graduated with university honors.

Due to a poor job market, however, Bob could not find employment when he graduated. Despite this, he persevered and eventually got a job in his chosen profession. His career started off slowly, and he faced a few setbacks early on, but he eventually hit his stride and was able to earn a comfortable living throughout his career.

Six months ago, at age 65, Bob retired. For the last six months, he has been struggling. He tries to stay active on a daily basis, but still finds himself in a bit of a funk, and is unable to find his way out.

"Something has got to change!" Bob finally mutters to himself. "I do not want to spend the next 20 to 30 years in absolute misery!" That's when Bob decides to seek professional help. Never one to rely on others, he initially struggles with this decision. However, the thought of living his life in abject misery and pain overwhelms his natural tendencies to go it alone.

Bob continues mulling over his thoughts as the therapist, Carol, enters the room.

———— ⊛ ————

Carol: Good morning, my name is Carol, and I am your therapist.

Bob: Good morning, Carol. My name is Bob.

Carol: How are you doing today, Bob?

Bob: Fine Carol, and you?

Carol: Fine, thank you. Well Bob, I have looked over your file, but I would like to hear from you, so why don't we start with you telling me why you came to see me?

Bob: Well, I'm 65 years old and I retired six months ago. Lately, something's been nagging at me. I get this empty feeling inside, though I'm not exactly sure why. I knew retirement was going to be a change, so I read books on it – you know, what to do, how to keep active, and all that. I thought I was ready for it. I figured I had adequately prepared.

When the day finally arrived, I was elated! No more having to get up at the crack of dawn each day. No more stress. No more meaningless, fruitless tasks to do throughout the day. No more office politics. No more late evenings at the office, taking work home with me, or entertaining clients. No more wasted time. From now on, I would get to do exactly what I wanted to do. My co-workers threw a big goodbye party for me, and it was great!

Carol: Sounds like you had a plan, which is a good start to any new journey, especially one that is based on retirement. So then what happened?

Bob: Well, the first couple weeks of retirement were great. Everything went exactly as planned. But then I began to experience something I never thought I would. I began to experience feelings of loneliness, boredom, sadness, emptiness, panic, and fear. I never expected to feel so many emotions all at the same time. It was as if the flood gates that were holding them back just burst open, and they all flooded in at once. Now I'm drowning in them. I wasn't prepared for that.

Carol: That is a fairly typical reaction. I hear this from a lot of people who come to see me, particularly from men and women who have had a career. Please continue.

Bob: Well, I'm very analytical, so one by one, I took each emotion and tried to figure out what was causing me to experience it.

Carol: Interesting approach. What did you find out?

Bob: Well, I won't bore you with all the details, but through my analysis, I discovered that certain elements of my previous life – my job, my co-workers, and even my employers – filled a great void for me.

Carol: How so?

Bob: Though I love having people around me, and love socializing, I've always been a bit of a loner. More exactly, I've always been a bit of an introvert. It was tough for me, but I eventually learned to deal with that by acting as if I were an extrovert … a social butterfly.

To do this, I relied on my job and all the social interactions that came with it. I relied on happy-hours, holiday parties, office relationships, and even office drama to keep me motivated and engaged. There always seemed to be something to keep me busy. Even when there wasn't, work was always there for me, sort of as a safety net.

Carol: What do you mean by safety net?

Bob: Work was there as a crutch, as a never-ending activity. Something I knew I could always rely on to keep me busy, keep me occupied, keep my mind off the fact that I was really an introvert who had trouble making friends, or interacting with people. Work was always there to fill the void.

Carol: I see.

Bob: I could work for hours on end; late into the evening on most days, in fact. Work really consumed me, leaving little time for anything else.

Carol: You must have really loved your work.

Bob: That's just the thing, I HATED EVERY GODDAMN MINUTE OF IT! I used to fantasize about what it would be like without a job; without that anchor around my neck. And I used to think about how great it would be when I finally got to retire.

Carol: And now you *are* retired. That has not brought you the relief you were looking for?

Bob: Not at all! In fact, just the opposite. It's made me feel downright depressed. I realized work was actually holding me together. Sure, I enjoyed fantasizing about being free from work, and having the freedom to do what I wanted, but I always knew, deep down, that this was just a fantasy, that I would never get a chance to realize my dream of being free, or any of my dreams for that matter. I knew my path had been pre-determined, and that freedom was not on that path.

As I say that out loud, it sounds depressing, but strangely, it provided me great comfort over the years.

Carol: Why was that?

Bob: Because it meant that no matter what happened, I would always be whole; I would always be fulfilled. I would never be left alone with only my thoughts to keep me company. It meant I never had to be afraid of facing loneliness and despair.

Carol: It sounds like you figured out how to make your life work in spite of your introverted personality. So what happened?

Bob: I retired. My job went away, and with it almost all the activities that kept me occupied for over 40 years. Suddenly, I had nothing but time on my hands. I was alone, with only my thoughts to keep me company, and I had no blasted idea what to do with myself! It was so damn depressing!

Carol: I see.

Bob: Yeah, it has not been a fun time for me. At first, I thought I could handle it. I said to myself, "Just do the things you like. That will keep you occupied, that will fill the void, that will distract you and keep your mind off your problems." So I started doing what I love to do – eating and drinking. I love good food and I love good wine. Problem was, I loved them a bit too much, and after a while, I started gaining weight and found myself getting drunk all the time.

My new "hobbies" actually made me feel more miserable, and I even started to become physically ill. The alcohol also depressed me after a while. All I wanted to do each day was lie in bed and watch TV, with wine and food, of course, which led to wanting to lie in bed more, eat more food, drink more wine, and watch more TV. That led to … well, you get the point.

Carol: Sounds like you went into a downward spiral.

Bob: Yeah, I sure did. It went on that way for a few months until I hit rock bottom. I started having chest pains, and ended up in the emergency room, fearful I'd had a heart attack. That's when I knew I didn't have the answer, that I couldn't find it by myself, and that I needed help.

Carol: So that's when you decided to come and see me?

Bob: Yes, sort of. I knew I needed help, but didn't know how to get it. So I started asking around. Fortunately for me, I still keep in touch with a few of my former co-workers. One of them retired a few years ago. When I told him my story, he said he had gone through something similar, and gave me your name. He told me that you specialize in helping people in my situation.

Carol: Yes, that is what I do. Actually, most of my clients come to me when they are in the same situation as you are. Most of them have recently retired, within the last five years or so. They also typically started out as you did, elated to finally be retired; excited to have nothing to do and nowhere to be. And, like you, they quickly found that not having anything to do actually created a big void in their lives, and that invariably led to feelings of emptiness, loneliness, fear, and depression.

Bob: Sounds very familiar. I'm a bit relieved to know I'm not alone. At least it's not just me who feels this way.

Carol: Not at all. Unfortunately, it is a common problem. I used to encounter it all the time in my previous line of work. That is why I became a therapist and started this practice.

Bob: So what did you do before you became a therapist?

Carol: I was a registered nurse, and I spent the majority of my career working at a skilled nursing facility in a retirement community. After that, I spent a decade as a geriatric in-home care specialist.

Bob: But I'm just recently retired. How does your experience help me? Most people you've cared for were quite a bit older than I am.

Carol: My experience, as well as my age, has allowed me to see the entire path that you are about to travel. Most people who have recently retired are able to engage in various external activities that help them fill the void retirement creates. They travel, volunteer, take up tennis or golf, go to exercise classes, and otherwise take advantage of all the activities that are available to people of active retirement age.

While this strategy is good, it relies on an individual's ability to engage in those types of external activities. When the individual starts to lose their ability to engage in those activities, that strategy falls apart, leaving them right back where they started – lonely, fearful, and depressed.

Bob: So you actually saw this happen to your patients?

Carol: Yes, and by the time I started to care for them, they had been lonely and depressed for so long, their health was actually beginning to decline. I saw this a lot when I was an in-home care specialist.

Bob: That must have been a tough experience for you.

Carol: Yes, it was tough. It greatly saddened me to see so many otherwise healthy individuals in premature decline.

Bob: So is that what led you into this line of work?

Carol: Well, not at first. After about 10 years as an in-home care specialist, I finally retired. I went through the exact same thing you are experiencing now. I had a great void in my life, which led me to experience sadness and depression. Except this time, it was for myself.

Bob: So what did you do?

Carol: I thought about it for a bit, then decided to use the techniques I had always used as a geriatric nurse. Except that now, I would apply them to my own life. Slowly, I formed those techniques into a set of steps to follow; sort of like mapping out a journey toward a destination. I began to follow this journey map, and found it worked wonderfully well for me. So well, in fact, that I recommended it to my close friends, and they all used it with similar success.

Bob: That's great, but how can your techniques and journey map help me? As I said, I'm quite a bit younger than you. At least I think I am. How old are you?

Carol: I am 85, but you have to remember, I developed the journey map and began to use it when I was 70 years of age. Also, most of my friends were in their late sixties or early seventies when they began to use it. You see, I wasn't as old when I began to use my journey map, and neither were my friends.

Bob: I'm sorry, that was rude of me.

Carol: Not at all. At 85, you lose all vanity regarding age … well, at least I do. However, you are correct in observing that you are several years younger than I was when I started on my own journey.

Bob: So doesn't that mean I should come and see you in a few years instead of now?

Carol: Well, you could, but I have found that the journey map works even better when it is started early. In fact, the earlier you begin, the better it will work for you. Some of my patients actually started on their journey BEFORE they retired, in a few instances, several years before.

Bob: Really! Why is that? Why does it work better the earlier you start, I mean?

Carol: Because my techniques work to keep you both happier and healthier *as* you age. If you can begin this journey when you are already relatively young and healthy, then the results you achieve will be even better.

Bob: So the journey works better if you start earlier. Okay, I guess I can see that, but *how* does it work?

Carol: It works based on what is already inside of you.

Bob: What does that mean?

Carol: Most people rely on external stimulation to achieve happiness – a cruise, an expensive vacation, dinner at a fancy restaurant, an expensive night out on the town, among other things. While this is effective, the happiness it brings is usually temporary, often disappearing when the external stimulation goes away.

A far better approach is to use what is inside of you to achieve happiness. Starting with what is inside of you results in sustained and long-lasting happiness.

Bob: Really? Using what's inside me to achieve happiness? That's hard to believe. And maybe a bit scary, depending on what's going on inside me.

Carol: I know, and most people who come to me feel that way at first. However, what they quickly discover is that they can make their own happiness, and they do not need tons of external stimulation to do that for them. In fact, that's the secret.

Bob: What's the secret?

Carol: Learning to rely on your inner self for your happiness. You see, using your inner self to create your own happiness is timeless, ageless, and you can use it wherever you are in life. You also no longer need to rely on external activities to make you happy, so you never lose the ability to experience happiness and fulfillment in life, no matter how old you get.

Bob: That sounds very appealing.

Carol: You do not have to be rich, either. Most of the external activities that we rely on to keep active cost money, sometimes a lot of money. If a person is rich, or at least well off, then they can engage in these types of activities. However, if a person is poor, then their options for engaging in traditional "keep active" activities are limited. Using your inner self to create your own happiness and fulfillment is absolutely free, which means this method is available to everyone.

Bob: Sounds great. So how do we begin?

Carol: We begin by discussing your goals. Let's talk about what it is that you wish to accomplish in these sessions. What outcomes are you looking for?

Bob: Good question! I've actually thought a lot about this over the last few months. In fact, the friend who recommended you also advised I should have definite goals in mind before coming to see you. He told me you would ask.

Carol: You came prepared, which is excellent. So, what *are* your goals?

Bob: Well … I just want to be happy. I also want to feel fulfilled – I mean, I've spent my entire life in the business world thinking I was successful, and I just don't feel any of that.

Carol: Happiness and fulfillment are good things to have in your life, indeed. Just so I am clear, could you please define each term for me? Let's start with happiness. What does happiness mean to you?

Bob: To me, happiness means being in a state of joy or contentment. It means being at ease in life, being carefree, being at peace. Is that the correct definition of happiness?

Carol: My definition of happiness does not matter. What matters is how *you* define it; what it means to *you*. What about health? Have you thought about how being healthy can contribute to your happiness?

Bob: Actually, I hadn't thought about health … but you're right … and I think that would benefit me … so let's add it to my goals.

Carol: So how would you define health?

Bob: I would say that health is a sound body and a sound mind; free from disease or ailment.

Carol: What do you mean by sound?

Bob: Vigorous, sturdy, vibrant, reliable, robust. It's funny, but I just realized how difficult it is to clearly define what appear to be simple terms.

Carol: That is one of the tricks of language. We use terms so frequently that we get careless with them, and their meanings become ambiguous. That is why I am asking you to define them for me. Let's move on to fulfillment, what does fulfillment mean to you?

Bob: To be fulfilled? Hmm. It means to be satisfied. To be complete, to be whole, to be content, to be finished, to be matured, to be fully accomplished. This definition is pretty close to my definition of happiness, isn't it?

Carol: The terms are close, but definitely distinct. If you feel fulfilled, then you are probably also happy, but you can be happy without feeling completely fulfilled.

Bob: Really?

Carol: Yes, as long as you have a definite plan to attain fulfillment, you can still be happy even though you have not yet achieved that fulfillment. Getting to fulfillment is a journey, and it occurs over a period of time, whereas happiness occurs at a specific point in time, and is a state of mind.

Bob: Okay, I can understand that. So now what?

Carol: Well, that is all the time we have for today, which is good because it gives both of us a chance to take a break and think about what came out of today's session.

Bob: Okay. I was just getting eager to hear what comes next, but you're right, perhaps I need a break too. So what happens next?

Carol: During this week, I will create a plan for you – a personal plan. The next time we meet, I will walk you through that plan and show you how you can use it to achieve your personal goals of happiness, health, and fulfillment.

Bob: Okay, I can hardly wait to see what you come up with! I'll see you next week.

———⊚———

Bob gets up from the chair and walks out of Carol's office. Carol does not get up, as she's already busy making notes from the session. On his way out, Bob stops by the reception desk to make his next appointment.

"How many more appointments should I make?" Bob asks the receptionist.

"It usually takes a few months for Carol to take her patients through the entire process," the receptionist remarks.

"Let's just set one appointment for now. Let's make it for next Tuesday at 3 PM," Bob says.

The receptionist looks at him for a moment without speaking. "But sir, Carol's appointment book fills up quickly, and you may not be able to find any time on her calendar if you only schedule one appointment at a time. In fact, you were lucky I had this slot available for you."

"I'll take my chances," Bob replies, as he turns and leaves the office. Despite her assurances, Bob is not convinced Carol can help him. He figures he will know that by the end of next week's session, then he will book the remaining appointments, if necessary.

The receptionist watches Bob walk out the door, shakes her head, and goes on about her business.

CHAPTER 2

Carol's Keys to Success

Carol sits quietly in her office, waiting for Bob to arrive for his appointment. She has spent the past week thinking about her initial conversation with Bob, reviewing her session notes, and crafting her plan to help him realize his stated goals. She is spending the last few minutes before their session putting together her final thoughts. Not wanting to break her concentration, she has arranged for her receptionist to escort Bob to her office once he arrives.

This meeting, the second patient meeting, is typically the most important one of all her therapy sessions. This is the meeting where Carol outlines the patient's journey and asks them to commit to it.

If Carol can reach the patient, if her message resonates with them, if they can see the possibilities of what might be, then they almost always commit to the journey. But, if Carol fails to reach the patient, if she cannot articulate herself properly, if she cannot get her message through, then all will be lost and the patient will most likely walk out, never to return.

The thought of losing a patient before the journey even begins scares and frustrates Carol. As a lifelong caregiver, it is her burning desire to help all who come to her. She hates to lose even one patient, and always blames herself if she cannot reach them.

"I know I can help Bob," Carol says to herself. "I just have to reach him."

Just as she finishes her thought, the receptionist pages Carol on her intercom. Bob has arrived. She tells the receptionist to show him in. A few seconds later, Carol's office door opens and in walks Bob. She smiles at him as he sits down in the chair opposite her.

Here we go! she thinks.

———⊛———

Carol: Hello Bob, how are you today?

Bob: I'm fine, Carol, and you?

Carol: I have been well, thank you.

Bob: What's on tap for today?

Carol: I have spent the time since our last meeting reviewing my notes and coming up with a plan to help you realize your goals. I would like to spend today's session reviewing that plan with you.

Bob: Sounds good. I'm interested to hear how you can help me.

Carol: Very good. But before we begin, I would like to check my understanding of the problem. As I understand it, you have just retired after a career of more than 40 years. Though initially excited about retirement, you quickly began to experience loneliness, boredom, sadness, emptiness, panic, fear, and depression.

You realized that retirement left a huge void in your life, which you tried to fill by developing new hobbies based on what you enjoy doing, which is eating rich food and drinking good wine. While this initially worked, you soon began to overdo it. You started eating too much food and drinking too much wine, leading you to rapidly gain weight and frequently become drunk. A few months of this routine landed you in the emergency room with chest pains. Afraid that your new hobbies would eventually kill you, you realized you needed to make changes and do things differently.

Bob: So far, so good.

Carol: Now, you are looking to achieve something greater. You want happiness, health, and fulfillment, but you do not know how to get them on your own, and you are looking for help. Am I correct?

Bob: You're spot on! So how can you help me?

Carol: By showing you how to unlock the doors to happiness, health, and fulfillment.

Bob: And how do I unlock them?

Carol: To unlock these doors, you will need the keys. There are three of them, and all three must be used to unlock each door. Just using one or two will not do; you must use all three keys on each door, or it will not open.

Bob: Okay, so what are the three keys?

Carol: I call them MIND, BODY, and SPIRIT, and they are all interrelated.

Bob: I've heard of mind, body, and spirit before, though not exactly in this context. And I've never heard them described as an interrelated set of keys. Could you tell me why each key is important, and how it relates to the other two?

Carol: I would be happy to. Before I begin, however, I think it would be useful to look at a diagram of the three keys so you can see how they relate to each other. There is a whiteboard in my office that I use when I need to illustrate something for patients. Just give me a second to draw you a simple diagram. It will help reinforce the idea as we discuss it.

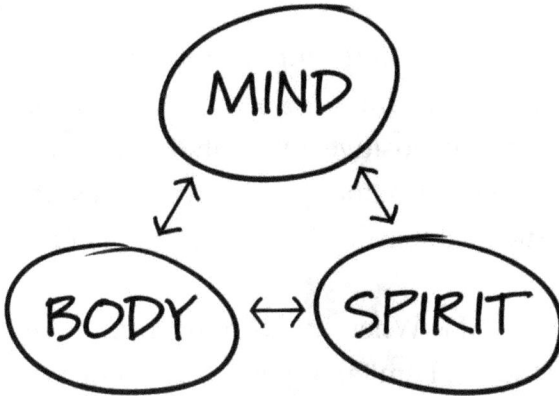

Carol: This diagram shows that mind, body, and spirit are inter-related keys. This is an important concept that I will speak about in a bit. But first, let's go through the keys one at a time.

The first key is MIND. Your mind is what allows you to be aware of your surroundings, and it helps you interpret everything you see and experience. Your mind also controls your thoughts and feelings, which can influence both your mental and emotional states, and can also impact your body – either positively or negatively.[1] So it is important that you control your thoughts and that you think positively. Positive thoughts lead to positive emotions and a healthier body, while negative thoughts lead to a negative emotional state, and can ultimately lead to an unhealthy body.

The next key is BODY. Your body is your physical structure, which includes your bones, your flesh, and your organs. Modern medicine has gotten quite good at maintaining the health of the human body. Unfortunately, many medical practitioners focus almost entirely on the body, ignoring both mind and spirit. It is true that a healthier body makes us feel better, which can positively influence both our emotional and mental states. What most practitioners miss, however, is that the reverse is also true; healthier, more positive thoughts cause a more positive emotional state, and can actually influence the health of the body more than medicine or medical procedure can alone.[2]

The last key is SPIRIT. When I talk about spirit, I am not talking in the religious sense, I am talking more about human spirit. You can therefore think of spirit as the seat of your emotions and your character. But for our purposes, it is the emotional aspect of spirit that we care about.

The state of your spirit is really about your emotional state. Having and maintaining a positive emotional state is important because it leads to a brighter outlook and more positive thoughts. A brighter outlook has actually been found to improve how both the mind and the body function.[3] So a positive emotional state leads to both a sounder mind and a sounder body.

Bob: This is all new to me … I'm not even sure I completely understand it. How does being in a positive emotional state lead to a brighter outlook?

Carol: It has to do with having a positive mental attitude. Being in a positive emotional state leads to a positive mental attitude, which leads to a brighter outlook.

Bob: So I think I get it, except for the part about mental attitude.

I mean, I understand what positive and negative mean, but what do you mean when you say that someone either has a positive or negative mental attitude?

Carol: Well, have you heard of the glass half full or glass half empty theory?

Bob: That explains it! So if I see the glass as half full, I have a positive mental attitude, and if I see the glass as half empty, I have a negative mental attitude?

Carol: Correct.

Bob: That all sounds good. But how do I get into a positive emotional state so I can get a positive mental attitude and attain this brighter outlook, as you call it?

Carol: That is what these sessions are about. If you are willing to give this some time, all will be revealed and explained.

Bob: Fair enough. So how do I use these keys?

Carol: You will learn how to use these keys over the course of our journey together, a journey we will be taking over the next few months. During this journey, we will be exploring the details behind each of these keys, and you will learn how to use them to unlock the doors to happiness, health, and fulfillment.

Bob: Sounds good.

Carol: One thing I must caution you on. Earlier, I told you that you must use all three keys to unlock each door, and that these keys are interrelated. That means you need to thoroughly understand how each key works. Do not try to skip over a key. You need all three for this process to work properly.

Think of it as a three-legged stool. All three legs are needed in order to make the stool stand. The stool would fall down if it only had one or two legs. Same principle. You need all three keys in order to make this process "stand."

Bob: Okay, I see what you're saying, and I won't skip. I'll learn about all three keys, I promise. What are the next steps?

Carol: Well, first you need to make three months' worth of appointments. Booking one appointment at a time will not do. I want to make sure you have a structure in place for the entire program. My schedule fills up quickly, and I want to make sure we have the same time blocked out each week. Routine and habit are important ingredients to this journey.

Bob: Don't worry, I'll set up three months' worth of appointments on my way out. I can do 3 PM on Tuesdays. Does that work?

Carol: Yes, I will pencil you in for 3 PM next Tuesday. Please see my receptionist on the way out to make that official, and to set up all of your appointments for the rest of our journey.

Bob: Will do. I'll see you next Tuesday at 3 PM. And thanks. It sounds like this will really help me; I'm looking forward to it.

———⊛———

Bob grins as he gets up from the chair and strolls out of Carol's office. Carol waits until Bob closes the door behind him before she breathes a sigh of relief. *Success!* she thinks. The second meeting has always been the toughest one for her, and she never really knows if her message has reached her patient or not. That is, until the meeting is actually over, and her patient commits to their journey.

Over the hump. Now the real work can begin. Carol is confident, but she has no idea what she's in for.

———⊛———

Bob stops by the reception desk and makes it official. He confirms his appointment for next week, and books three months' worth of appointments, all for Tuesdays at 3 PM. Bob struts out of the office with a smile on his face and a spring in his step, something he had never expected to experience just one short week ago.

But somewhere in the back of his mind, he can't help thinking that he feels better just because he now has something each week to look forward to. Deep down, he knows this "social contact" is only partly replacing what he's lost, and that seeing a therapist may not be the answer. But he's willing to give it a try, even if it's only a temporary fix, which he vaguely fears it might be.

CHAPTER 3

⌒

Spirit: Part I

Carol is excited. She has been looking forward to this meeting with Bob all week. Here is where the journey finally begins. Here is where she begins to help patients transform their lives. Carol loves to make a positive difference in her patients' lives, which is why she started her practice when she was in her mid-seventies, and it's the reason she continues her work today, well into her mid-eighties. She loves her work so much, in fact, that she doesn't plan on retiring anytime soon.

———@———

It's Tuesday at 3 PM, and Bob is sitting in the waiting room, eagerly anticipating his upcoming session. Suddenly, he sees Carol emerge from her office. Bob stands up and Carol ushers him in. He takes his usual seat across from her, and they are ready to begin.

———@———

Carol: Hello Bob, how are you today?

Bob: Fine Carol, and you?

Carol: I am well, thank you for asking.

Bob: What's on tap for today?

Carol: As you recall, there are three keys that unlock the doors to happiness, health, and fulfillment. These three keys are Mind, Body, and Spirit. Today, we are going to begin our journey by talking about SPIRIT.

Bob: You're starting with Spirit? Last time, you started with Mind, so I thought you would start there.

Carol: All three keys are interrelated and influence each other, so it really does not matter where we start. However, I find that going through Spirit first can be very enlightening for my patients. I also find that it is easier for patients to understand the remaining two keys if we cover Spirit first.

Bob: Okay, let's start with Spirit then.

Carol: Very good. Just to keep us grounded and focused, I would like to briefly re-state the problem. You have just retired after a career of over 40 years. Though initially excited, you quickly began to experience loneliness, boredom, sadness, emptiness, panic, fear, and depression. You realized that retirement left a huge void in your life. Attempts to fill this void by yourself were ultimately unsuccessful, and you realized you needed help to achieve your goals of happiness, health, and fulfillment.

Bob: Yes, that's my problem ... That's why I'm here.

Carol: Okay, so let's proceed to talk about Spirit. As I said in our last session, when I talk about Spirit, I am talking about your emotional state. "Keeping your spirits up," as the saying goes. Your emotional state influences your overall wellbeing. A positive emotional state leads to a positive mental attitude and ultimately to a healthier body, while a negative emotional state leads to a negative mental attitude, which has a negative impact on the body.[4]

Bob: Sounds too simple. There's got to be more to it than that.

Carol: It is fairly straightforward; there is no magic to it. How our bodies react to stress and other negative forces has been scientifically measured.

Bob: Okay... so how can I go about achieving this positive emotional state that you say is so important?

Carol: In my experience, there are eight techniques that, when used diligently, help a person to achieve a positive emotional state. I will list them out for you, then we can discuss each one in more detail.

1. Be thankful for what you have
2. Surround yourself with family
3. Have close friends, but choose them wisely
4. Be happy for others' good fortune
5. Look at the beauty of nature around you
6. Do something for someone else
7. Do the things you enjoy doing
8. Find some way to release your frustrations

Bob: I don't know, Carol. This sounds like quackery to me! I don't see how merely doing these things can lead to happiness, health, and fulfillment.

Carol: Could you elaborate on your comment a bit more?

Bob: I'm sorry. I'm a very analytical person, and I just can't believe that merely thinking positive thoughts and putting on rose-colored glasses will really change anything. Isn't our destiny set in stone anyway? Isn't our path pre-determined for us? What choice do we have but to accept our fate?

Sure, I can see how doing these things might improve my emotional state, but I can't see how they will improve my health, or change anything of significance! I would just be deluding myself into believing I can change things when I know damn well that I can't. So what's the point of even bothering with any of this nonsense?

Carol: I sense that you are having a strong reaction to this. Not totally unexpected, but you seemed to be quite enthusiastic last week when you left my office. What changed?

Bob: I got to thinking about it, and I reminded myself that the best any of us can hope to do is to get through life as best as possible, and that the choices we make don't really have anything to do with how happy or sad we are. Most of our lives happen purely by chance, and no amount of effort on anyone's part can change that fact.

If we're fortunate enough to be born into wealth, then we're happy, but most of us are not that fortunate. Most of us were born into modest circumstances and live meager lives filled with misery, and there's not one damn thing any of us can do to change that. We all just have to deal with the hand that we're dealt, which is unfair, but that's the way it is. Life's a kick in the teeth for most of us.

Carol: There are countless rich people who are miserable, and plenty of less fortunate people who are happy. While you are correct that a child cannot influence the environment they are born into, and that environment has a very big influence on a person's outlook on life, people do have choices. In fact, people have more power to choose than they think. Life is really all about choices, and the choices people make always influence their outcomes.

Bob: That may be true – that there are unhappy rich people and happy poor ones, but as for the rest of it, I don't buy it!

Carol: It's true. Choice influences outcome. It is all about cause and effect. You are analytical, so you must believe in the principle of cause and effect – that every effect has a corresponding cause.

Bob: I do, but I don't see how we have any influence over cause.

Carol: The choices we make always cause something to happen, which will always lead to an effect. That effect can be either positive or negative – a good outcome or a bad one. Regardless of outcome, the point is that each and every cause will result in an effect, and each effect has a corresponding cause. It is a natural law of the universe.

Bob: Okay, I'm beginning to see your point, but I still don't see what any of this has to do with elevating my emotional state.

Carol: Well, positive thoughts cause positive emotions, and positive emotions lead to the effect of a positive emotional state. Put another way, positive thoughts cause you to "keep your spirits up," which is the resulting effect. For example, when you think about someone you love, maybe even your dog, your brain creates endorphins, chemicals which have been scientifically measured and proven to elevate your mood.[5,6] So positive thoughts cause your brain to release endorphins, which has the effect of putting you into a positive emotional state.

Bob: Okay, now I see what you're saying. But I still need more details. I'm not sure what to do with this list of eight things you just gave me.

Carol: Fair enough. I will go into more detail on each item, one at a time. Let's start with item one – **Be thankful for what you have**.

Bob: Okay, tell me why that's important. How does that work to help me unlock the doors to happiness, health, and fulfillment?

Carol: You will be much more pleased with your life if you are thankful for what you have. Just like thinking about someone you love, being thankful for what you have puts you into a positive emotional state. What is something you are thankful for?

Bob: Does ice cream count?

Carol: Yes, ice cream counts. That is, if you have it, or have the ability to buy it.

Bob: I don't have it, but I know a place where I can buy it.

Carol: Why are you smiling?

Bob: Because just thinking about that ice cream cone I'm going to get when I leave here is making me happy.

Carol: Good. Now you get it. Being thankful for what you have puts you into a positive emotional state, and helps you unlock the doors to happiness, health, and fulfillment. Alternatively, nothing puts you into a negative emotional state, and prevents you from unlocking those doors, faster than focusing on what you do not have.

Bob: What do you mean?

Carol: Let's continue with your ice cream example. Suppose the ice cream parlor you go to this evening is out of your favorite flavor?

Bob: If that's the case, then I'll be very upset and disappointed that I can't get what I want.

Carol: Do you like only one flavor of ice cream, or could you choose another flavor?

Bob: I like most flavors of ice cream, so I guess I could pick another flavor that would make me happy.

Carol: So, focusing on an ice cream flavor that you cannot get makes you upset and disappointed, but focusing on a flavor that you can get makes you much happier.

Bob: Okay, I see that, but what's your point?

Carol: Different focuses put you into different emotional states. When you focus on what you do not have, that puts you into a negative emotional state. However, if you learn to focus on what you do have, then that puts you into a positive emotional state. The point is to focus on what you have, rather than on what you do not.

Bob: Okay, I understand, but ice cream is such a small thing. I mean, I don't have millions of dollars or a lot of expensive stuff in my life to be thankful for. So what can I do?

Carol: Let me give you an example. One that will illustrate how you can *choose* to be thankful for what you have, no matter what environment you were born into, or how much money you have or don't have.

I was born into a middle-class family. While I had a very loving mother and father, we did not have much money. There was no such thing as a two-income family like there is today. Back then, fathers were the breadwinners, and mothers stayed at home. Because of this, my parents did not have enough money to buy me a bike, or even roller skates.

All the families in our neighborhood were in the same situation, all struggling to make ends meet. Thankfully, we lived in a small tight-knit community where everyone, including the children, knew each other, so it was relatively easy for me to make friends. On most days, all the children in our neighborhood would play street games, which did not require the use of any expensive or elaborate toys – which none of us had anyway.

Regardless of how much money our parents did or did not have, we all had ropes to jump, chalk to make hopscotch games, and balls to throw. We were thankful for the neighborhood we lived in, thankful for the neighbors we knew, and thankful for the toys that we *did have* to play with. At no time did we focus on what we did not have, and we all felt happy, healthy, and fulfilled.

Bob: That's quite a story, but I'm not sure I get your point.

Carol: The point is that you have a choice. With everything you have, and with every decision you make, you choose how to be: grateful or ungrateful, happy or sad, joyful or angry, loving or hateful.

Bob: What do you mean?

Carol: I had a modest upbringing, and I did not have a lot of material things, yet I was very happy as a child. Rather than focusing on what I did not have, which would have caused me to feel the negative emotions of jealousy, envy, and hate, I chose to be thankful for what I had, which gave me a more positive outlook on life, and put me into a positive emotional state.

Bob: I see.

Carol: What's more, these negative emotions can do more damage than you might imagine. Your emotional state affects your mental state. A negative emotional state leads to a negative mental state, which can cause a defeatist attitude. It can lead you to live your life in constant envy of everyone else; jealous of what they have that you do not. It can also leave you with feelings of helplessness, hopelessness, and want.

If that thinking persists long enough, it could actually negatively affect your body by causing you stress and anxiety, which could lead to things such as ulcers or even a nervous breakdown.[7]

Bob: Okay, that clarifies it. So now I get how negative emotions and a negative emotional state could affect my happiness, my health, and could leave me feeling unfulfilled. But what can I do about it?

Carol: I want you to list out at least 10 things you have that you are thankful for. More is better, but list at least 10 things.

Bob: How will that help?

Carol: Physically seeing a list of the things you have that you are thankful for will start to put you into a positive emotional state, just like when you thought about the ice cream cone. Please make this list and be ready to discuss it the next time we meet.

Bob: Okay, I'll give it a try. What's next?

Carol: The next thing you can do to put yourself into a positive emotional state is to **surround yourself with family**.

Bob: Why is that important? How does surrounding myself with family help me achieve my goals?

Carol: When you surround yourself with family, you are surrounding yourself with people who love you. In addition to being a very powerful positive emotion, love also brings about positive feelings such as joy, comfort, and contentment. And positive feelings like these are what put you into a positive emotional state, which will ultimately help you achieve your goals.

Bob: So you're saying it's important to surround myself with people who love me, but what if I'm estranged from my family?

Carol: Estrangement creates tension, drama, and bad feelings; all of which ultimately lead to a negative emotional state. Work to repair those relationships so they will nourish you with positive, rather than negative, energy.

Bob: So if I'm estranged from my family, I need to repair my relationships with them BEFORE I can unlock the doors to happiness, health, and fulfillment?

Carol: You do not need to have perfect relationships with your family members in order to reach your goals, and you should not let that become an excuse for why you are not happy, healthy, and fulfilled. Ideally, you will want to repair strained relationships with family members, as this will yield the best results for you. However, this will take time and effort on your part, and it may be a while until you see tangible results.

Bob: I'm not sure I follow you.

Carol: Think of it as tending a garden. Tending a garden requires a lot of initial effort – cultivating the soil, planting the seeds, watering the ground, and so forth. And for several weeks afterward, you see no results. However, if you keep up your effort, over time, the garden will begin to produce fruits and vegetables. It is the same with repairing relationships. You will need to put in time and effort up front, and at first, you may not see any results. Over time, however, your efforts will begin to bear fruit.

Bob: I see, so I need to put in a lot of time and effort at the start?

Carol: Not just at the start. Like gardening, relationships require continuous effort. If you stop watering your garden, the seedlings will stop growing. The same is true with relationships. If you stop putting in the time and effort, then they will stop growing.

Bob: Okay, so assuming I have relationship issues with my family, and that repairing them will take some time, then who should I surround myself with in the meantime?

Carol: Surround yourself with people who love you. Family is not limited to only blood relatives. Family can also be adopted family members; people you have come to think of as family. For instance, we may call someone who is close to the family Aunt Linda or Uncle Willy even though they are not actually blood relatives. The most important thing is to surround yourself with positive emotions and feelings, ones which put you into a positive emotional state.

Bob: But it's just so hard today. Many of my family members, even my so-called adopted ones, have either moved away or travel so much that I hardly see them anymore.

Carol: I understand, and I would be lying if I said this was not a real issue. Fortunately, the Internet and cell phones help us to keep in touch. Though this is not as satisfying as being together, it does keep us connected.

Bob: I'm kind of old fashioned. I like talking to people in person, or keeping in touch through letters. Getting a response to a letter is like getting a present in the mail – it gives me something to look forward to.

Carol: How you choose to communicate is ultimately up to you, but keeping in touch with family any way you can will ultimately put you into a positive emotional state.

Bob: Okay, so how do I make use of this technique?

Carol: Make a list of your family members. This list can include either blood relatives, adopted family, or both. Next to the name of each family member, write the current state of your relationship with them. For example, is your relationship with them good, or is it strained? How close do you currently feel to them, very close or very distant? How do you feel emotionally when you think of them? Do you feel happy, or angry, or sad?

If you are not on good terms with a particular family member, it will also help to write down what caused the relationship to become strained. This will give you a perspective that might prove helpful when you begin to repair the relationship.

Bob: Okay, I can see why writing down what caused my family

relationships to become strained would be helpful, but what's the reason for listing out all the emotions?

Carol: The point of this exercise, and all other Spirit exercises, is to help you generate positive emotions, which put you into a positive emotional state. But you also want to avoid negative emotions, which will do just the opposite. Therefore, you want to know exactly what emotions you experience when you think of each family member, and whether they are positive or negative ones. Writing them down gives you the opportunity to observe the specific emotions that each family member causes you to feel. It will also help you identify family relationships that need to be repaired.

Bob: Okay, I'll make the list, but then how do I use it?

Carol: First, make the list, then we can talk about what to do with it.

Bob: Okay, fair enough. What's next?

Carol: We just talked about the importance of surrounding yourself with family. The next technique, **have close friends**, builds on that.

Bob: Okay, why's that important, and how does it help me achieve my goals?

Carol: Like family, having close friends who love you can do wonders to lift your spirits. Close friends who love you can put you into a very positive emotional state; they are usually non-judgmental, supportive, and make you feel good about yourself.

Bob: I'm not sure I understand how having close friends will lift my spirits.

Carol: As human beings, we all have a need to belong, be it to an entire community, or to just a small group. For example, think of the time you were in high school. Remember the high school "cliques" that certain kids were a part of?

Bob: I do. Very well, in fact.

Carol: You can also extend this example to social clubs and professional organizations. These are all groups that fulfill a basic human need – the need to belong. Your former job is another example. Even though you did not like your job, you most likely looked forward to "belonging" to a company of people, which probably gave you a purpose, and made you feel needed.

Bob: Okay, so I felt needed, so what?

Carol: We all need to be needed. It gives us our sense of personal worth. Just knowing that there is a group of people out there who find it valuable to associate with us makes us feel valued and needed.

Bob: Okay, I get it … I think. The way you used my job as an example sort of made a light bulb go off in my head. So belonging to a community, group, or organization makes us feel needed and lifts our spirits. But I'm not making the connection between belonging to a group and having close friends.

Carol: Well, you and your close friends form another type of group, albeit one that is self-selected.

Bob: Oh, now I see.

Carol: And it's not just feeling needed that lifts your spirits. Close friendships add a strong emotional component as well, namely love, and the feeling of acceptance that comes with it. As I have already mentioned, love is a very powerful emotion, one of the most powerful emotions in all of humanity. And nothing elevates a person's emotional state more quickly than when they are loved by someone.

Bob: So I can see how positive emotions elevate someone's Spirit, but how do they impact Mind and Body?

Carol: We will talk in detail about that during the course of our sessions. But you may find it interesting to know that scientific research is starting to identify the impact emotions have on both the mind and body. For example, one study has identified how various emotionally charged words cause different physical reactions in the body, such as increased heart rate, more rapid breathing, or increased brain activity.[8]

Bob: Okay, I'm starting to see how this all connects now, and I get the importance of having close friends. I think we can move on.

Carol: Before we do, I want to impress upon you the importance of choosing your close friends wisely.

Bob: What do you mean by that?

Carol: Good friends, true friends, can do wonders to elevate your spirits. They bring joy and happiness with them wherever they go. However, make sure to avoid people who bring you down. Avoid people who mope around all day and complain.

Bob: I'm not sure I understand. Do you have an example?

Carol: Sure. Think about Eeyore, the donkey in the *Winnie the Pooh* books.[9] Eeyore is always depressed; he always has a "Woe is me" response when anyone asks him how he is doing. The world is full of human Eeyores, people who complain all the time, about anything and everything.

As a geriatric nurse, I used to see some patients do nothing but sit around and complain about their ailments all day long. Even though I was not part of their group, just hearing those conversations put me in a bad mood.

But it was even worse. Without knowing it, each member of that group had a hand in depressing themselves, and negatively affecting each other's emotional, mental, and physical states. By complaining about their ailments, they were actually perpetuating them.

Bob: Okay, now I get it. But what can I do about it?

Carol: Surround yourself with people who bring you joy and happiness, people who lift you up rather than bring you down.

Bob: What do you mean?

Carol: I will give you an example from my own life to illustrate. In my case, I am extremely blessed to have close friendships. I met most of my friends in church or in my neighborhood. My friends are truly special; they are never unkind, critical, or negative, and from the moment I met them, I knew they would be great friends.

Bob: I see.

Carol: Also, good friends stand by you, through both difficult and good times. It is very comforting to know that your friends are always there for you; always there to lean on when you need them. That is a great feeling to have, and it quickly puts you into a positive emotional state.

Bob: Okay, so I get that, but how do I handle the Eeyores?

Carol: Avoid them. People like that will do nothing but cause you stress, anxiety, and despair, which will put you into a negative emotional state, lead to a chronically negative frame of mind, and could adversely affect you physically by causing you an ulcer, high blood pressure, or worse. We will talk more about how to avoid Eeyores throughout our sessions, but for now, just know that you should avoid them at all costs.

Bob: Okay, so how do I use this technique?

Carol: First, I want you to do some homework for me. Take the list of family members that you compiled as part of the second technique – **Surround yourself with family**, and add the names of your close friends. Now for each person on your updated list, I want you to mark whether they are an Eeyore. We will discuss how you can use that list during our next session.

Bob: Okay, looks like we're making some progress. What's next?

Carol: The next thing you can do to lift your spirits is to **be happy for others' good fortune**.

Bob: Be happy for others? I thought the point was to put ME into a positive emotional state?

Carol: It is. This technique works by getting YOU to be happy, which puts you into a positive emotional state.

Bob: But I'm not being happy for me, I'm being happy for some-one else.

Carol: The point of this exercise is to get YOU to be happy, peri-od. It does not matter *what* you are happy about; what matters is that you *are* happy about *something*. Also remember, what goes around comes around. Stated another way, you get what you give, but you must give first. Read Emerson's "Compensation," it is a fascinating essay that goes into great detail on this subject.[10]

Bob: So you're saying that, by being happy for someone else, they will also be happy for me?

Carol: People tend to mirror the emotions you display towards them, so this is usually the case. In addition, your emotions tend to mirror your thoughts, so positive thoughts lead to positive emotions. By merely expressing happiness for someone else, you will generally receive a happy feeling as a result, even if the per-son you are happy for does not immediately return the feeling.

Bob: Okay, I understand the theory, but how do I apply this in practice?

Carol: Applying this technique is quite simple. Just let others know you are happy for them. For example, there is great joy in seeing family members and friends have good things happen to them. Perhaps it is a salary increase, a job promotion, being able to buy a house, inheriting money, luck in the stock market, or a new baby. Whatever it is, let them know you are happy for them, and ask if you can tell others about their good fortune.

Bob: I see.

Carol: And you do not need to limit this to family and friends. If a child in your neighborhood gets a new bicycle, tell them how happy you are to see them riding it. Applying this technique is really just that easy.

Bob: But what if I don't have good fortune? And what if I'm actually envious or jealous of others' good fortunes?

Carol: Forget about the material things others have that you do not. Those thoughts only invite the negative emotions of jealousy, envy, hatred, and want. Remember, you are trying to put yourself into a positive emotional state.

Bob: Okay, but don't I have to be happy for myself first?

Carol: Most people believe they must be happy for themselves BEFORE they can be happy for others. The truth is, you can become happy for yourself BY being happy for others. Just like a mirror, when you give happiness to someone, it gets reflected back at you.

Bob: Sounds a bit strange. I'm not sure I buy it.

Carol: Then I want you to try a little experiment for me. Think of the last time someone you deeply cared for called to tell you about something good that happened to them. How did their news make you feel?

Bob: I was happy for them … Okay, now I see what you mean.

Carol: I am glad you see the humor in that little example.

Bob: Yeah, it was cute. So what's next? I mean, how do I use this technique?

Carol: First, I have a homework assignment for you. I want you to take the list of family and friends you started and build on it. For each person on your list, I want you to think of something good that has happened to them and write that next to their name. I will show you how to use this list during our next session.

Bob: Okay, I'll make the list, then you can show me how to use it. What's next?

Carol: Another thing you can do to elevate your spirits is to **look at the beauty of nature around you.**

Bob: How does that help?

Carol: Have you ever looked up at the stars on a clear night, or watched the sunset?

Bob: No.

Carol: How about watching the sunrise, or taking a walk on a crisp autumn morning and marveling at the color of the leaves as they turn?

Bob: I do like fall; it's my favorite time of year. I like the temperature of the air, and I enjoy watching the leaves change color.

Carol: And how does that make you feel?

Bob: I don't know. Alive, I guess.

Carol: No, I want you to really think about this for a moment without answering me.

Bob: … Okay, I've thought about it.

Carol: Good, now tell me all the things that you love about fall, and how they make you feel.

Bob: I love the harvest season, going apple picking, finding the perfect pumpkins for the front of the house. I love going to the wineries in California and Oregon for all the harvest celebration dinners. I love all the foods that come with the fall season.

Carol: And now that you are really thinking of everything you enjoy about the fall season, how do you feel?

Bob: I feel happy. I feel kind of joyful in fact.

Carol: I can see that on your face, and you also just answered your own question.

Bob: What do you mean?

Carol: Everything about fall that you just described is part of nature. The colors on the leaves, the cool nip in the air, the apples, and the pumpkins. Even the wine dinners that you so love, they all come from nature's bounty.

All these things, by your own admission, make you happy. By looking at the beauty of nature around you, you have automatically put yourself into a positive emotional state without even realizing it.

Bob: I never thought of it like that … But I thought all of your techniques were cost-free. Don't the wine dinners cost money?

Carol: Well, in some instances, yes, you *can* spend money to marvel at the beauty of nature, like taking an Alaskan cruise, going on a guided safari in Africa, or spending money on an upscale harvest dinner. However, these are not the only ways to marvel at the beauty of nature. There are many ways to do that without spending any money at all.

Bob: Name one.

Carol: Actually, you already named one. You mentioned that you like going for walks in the fall and watching the leaves changing colors. What does that cost you?

Bob: I see your point.

Carol: I'll give you another example. Recently, I stayed at my niece's home for about six weeks while on vacation. My niece is a naturalist who enjoys all that nature has to offer. She was raising butterflies at the time, and she had three butterfly cages – three caterpillars in each one. For those six weeks, I watched each day as those caterpillars went through their transition into butterflies. It was a marvel to watch. To me, there is nothing more beautiful than seeing a butterfly developing; it is an amazing miracle.

Bob: I'm not into butterflies.

Carol: Do you like to garden? I find that just planting a dry seed in soil, nurturing it with water and sunlight, then seeing it germinate and begin to grow out of its protective covering, is miraculous. It soon becomes a seedling, and then a thriving plant. It is a joy to watch, and it costs almost nothing, just a few cents for a package of seeds.

Bob: I'm not really into gardening, either.

Carol: That is quite okay. This actually leads me to another homework assignment I have for you. You actually already started this one, but I want you to complete it before our next session.

Bob: What's that? What did I start, and what do I need to complete?

Carol: I want you to write down at least 10 things that you find beautiful in nature. You already started this list when you gave me the things you enjoy about fall – the changing of the leaves, the apple picking, the harvest dinners. Complete that list before our next session.

Bob: Okay, then what?

Carol: Just like the other lists you are making, I will show you how to use it the next time we meet.

Bob: Can't you show me now?

Carol: We still have a lot of ground to cover this week, so I will show you next week.

Bob: Okay, then let's keep going. What's next?

Carol: The next technique I have for lifting your spirits is to **do something for someone else**.

Bob: So with this technique, you're telling me that *before* I can feel good about myself I've got to help others?

Carol: I would state it another way. I would say that this technique allows you to feel good about yourself *by* helping others.

Bob: Fair enough.

Carol: This goes back to the Law of Compensation. In his essay, Emerson states that everything has a cost, and that cost and income are really just two sides of the same coin.[11] Therefore, you will be justly compensated for every act you perform, or every cost you incur. In other words, what goes around comes around.

Bob: Okay, I think I understand. So tell me more.

Carol: It is through the act of giving to others – Doing something good for your neighbor. Being a good Samaritan. Contributing to society in some small way – that you will achieve a good feeling about yourself.

Bob: But how does that work?

Carol: Well, as the Law of Compensation states, you get what you give. More precisely, you get *back* what you give, sometimes many times over.

Bob: I'm not sure I'm following you.

Carol: Think about the last time you did something for someone else. How did that make you feel?

Bob: I can't remember the last time I did something for someone else.

Carol: I am sure you have. Let me see if I can help you to remember. Have you ever walked into a busy convenience store that was full of people?

Bob: Of course, I was just in one earlier this week. It was so busy; people constantly coming and going.

Carol: And when you left, did you hold the door for the person behind you?

Bob: Well, yeah. I always try to do that.

Carol: And how did that make you feel?

Bob: Good, I guess. They said thank you to me and everything. It's always nice to have your efforts acknowledged by someone else.

Carol: Okay good, let's continue along this line. In that same convenience store, have you ever forgotten to hold the door for someone as you left?

Bob: Admittedly yes, though it wasn't intentional. It'd been a while since I'd been in that particular store, and I guess I just got lost in my thoughts and forgot that people were constantly coming and going. Anyway, I forgot to hold the door a couple of times.

Carol: And how did that make you feel?

Bob: I felt selfish and thoughtless, as if I only cared about myself.

Carol: That example illustrates my point.

Bob: What point?

Carol: Doing something for someone else, no matter how minor, provides us with good feelings, putting us into a positive emotional state. In that convenience store, just as the Law of Compensation states, you got what you gave. You held the door for someone else, and they repaid you by saying thank you, which made you feel good. Said another way, they paid you for your act of holding the door with good feelings.

Bob: Huh ... I never thought of it that way.

Carol: It works the other way, too. When you forgot to hold the door, when you forgot to do something for someone else, when you were selfish and thought only of yourself, your act was repaid, but this time you were repaid with bad feelings.

Bob: Interesting. So should I always expect to be repaid for my actions?

Carol: Yes, you should. And sometimes, your kindness will be repaid several times over. A compounding effect, if you will.

Bob: What do you mean?

Carol: Let me give you an example. I usually buy fresh fruits and vegetables at a local produce market. They sell their food for much less than the regular markets do, so I am able to share half of what I buy with my neighbors, who repay my kindness by mowing my lawn and shoveling my walkway when it snows. If I had to pay for those services, it would cost me 10 times more than the few dollars I spend for the fruits and vegetables I "give away." So, not only am I compensated by the gratitude and appreciation my neighbors give to me, but I am also compensated with services that would have cost me a lot of money if I had to pay for them.

Bob: Okay, now I see how both the Law of Compensation and the compounding effect work.

Carol: Good. I need to give you a word of caution, however. Do not expect to be compensated directly by the person you performed the good deed for. While you may indeed be compensated directly and immediately for your actions, this is not guaranteed. However, the Law of Compensation states that you *will* eventually be compensated for your actions, just not necessarily right away.

Bob: Okay, I think I finally understand this technique now. So how do I use it?

Carol: Before I show you that, I have another homework assignment for you. I want you to make a list of at least 10 things you have done for someone else. These things could either be in the recent or distant past. Next to each item, write down how that good deed made you feel, and how you were compensated for it. Remember, your compensation does not necessarily come from the person you did the good deed for, nor does it necessarily immediately follow that good deed. Compensation can come days, months, or even years afterward.

Bob: That might be tough. What if I don't know how I was compensated?

Carol: That's okay. If you do not recognize how you were compensated for a specific action, just leave a blank next to it. However, for each action on your list, do write down how it made you feel. That part is important.

Bob: Okay, I'll give it a try. What's next?

Carol: **Do the things you enjoy doing**.

Bob: That one's easy. I can see how doing something that I enjoy leads to happiness.

Carol: Yes, this one is kind of obvious. In fact, if you hyphenate the word en-joy, you will see that joy is the second part of the word.

Bob: Okay, so no need to elaborate on this one. Just give me the exercise I need to do, and let's move on to the last technique.

Carol: I know you think we can skip over this technique, but it is important that we discuss it.

Bob: Why? This one seems so obvious, what more can you say?

Carol: I know this seems intuitive, and it is, so I am sure it will surprise you to learn that most people don't do the things they enjoy doing. In fact, they do exactly the opposite.

Bob: What do you mean?

Carol: Most people stay at miserable jobs, put up with lousy relationships and rebellious kids, get stuck in cycles of endless chores and "honey-do" lists, and so forth. All because they think they have no choice.

Bob: I can relate. I did that for many years, I felt like I had no choice. I felt compelled to do the things I did. Even though I hated my job, I had to support my family, raise my kids, and put them through school. My wife and I fought all the time, but we stayed married for the sake of the kids. My kids were rebellious teens – entitled and ungrateful. But I put them through school anyway. Like I said, I felt like I had no choice.

But all that's over now. I'm retired, my wife passed away a few years ago, and my kids all graduated college and moved away. They're busy with their own lives now, so I rarely hear from them. So that means now I'm free to do what I want. So what's the problem?

Carol: It may be that you have been doing the things you hate to do for so long that they have become a habit. And the longer you have a habit, the harder it is to break. As the saying goes, old habits die hard, and this particular bad habit can have serious negative consequences.

Doing things you hate to do increases your stress level, makes you miserable, and generally puts you into a negative emotional state. If this continues for a prolonged period, the stress and anxiety caused by constantly doing activities you hate can actually cause physical ailments, such as ulcers, high blood pressure, or weight gain. And, in the most severe case, could land you in the hospital with a stroke or heart attack.

Bob: So I get that doing unpleasant things causes me anxiety and stress, but I don't understand how this has become a bad habit that I need to consciously break.

Carol: Let me state it another way. It is human nature to resist change. We all tend to stay in our comfort zones, where we feel safe and protected. Most of us spend the majority of our lives doing what we do not want to do because we think we must. We believe we need to go to work, pay the bills, send the kids to college, mow the lawn, and so on. And we do this for so long that this behavior becomes a well-ingrained habit. We become used to it; it becomes familiar to us.

We are so used to doing things a certain way that, once we retire and finally do have a choice, many of us don't have any idea what to do. So we end up taking the path of least resistance. We do nothing; we sit on the couch and watch TV to pass the time. It is this bad habit that you need to consciously break.

Bob: But I do need to pay the bills and mow the lawn, among other things.

Carol: There are some chores that you will still need, or want, to do – like mowing the lawn, taking out the trash, or even going to the dentist. However, the point is to try and balance the things you have to do with the things you enjoy doing. We will address this as part of your next homework assignment.

Bob: Which is?

Carol: Make a list of at least 10 things you enjoy doing. You can put anything on this list, whether you have done it yet or not. You might include only enjoyable things you have done in the past, but you can also include things you have not done yet, but might enjoy doing in the future.

Bob: This seems like a strange question, but what about sex? Can I include sex as one of the activities I enjoy?

Carol: Of course, if you so choose. But why do you even feel that you have to ask if it is okay to put sexual activity on your list? After all, it is *your* list. You are the one who decides what is relevant and important, not me.

Bob: I don't know. I guess it's because I've always thought of sex as a vice – somewhat of a taboo topic, more so as I get older.

Carol: Well, you are not alone in thinking that way. The fact is, a lot of people are uncomfortable talking about sexual activity, especially as they age. Even some people in the medical profession are not comfortable discussing sexual activity with their older patients. However, research is beginning to show the importance of sexual activity in maintaining an elevated mood, and a higher quality of life as we age.[12]

Bob: So sex actually promotes an elevated emotional state, and can lead to happiness, health, and fulfillment?

Carol: Simply having sex does not contribute to lasting fulfillment. While it is true that the physical act of sex does produce good feelings, mainly through the release of endorphins that are produced by the brain during sex, the effect is short term in nature. Research has shown a correlation between feeling emotionally close to your partner during sex and a greater enjoyment of life.[13] It is this emotional connection, in conjunction with sex, that has the greatest impact on achieving long-term fulfillment.

Bob: I see, so I shouldn't just go to a bar and pick up a different woman every night, then? It sounds like that won't lead to lasting fulfillment. So, what should I do if I want romance in my life?

Carol: It is ultimately up to you how and where you choose to meet your potential partner. However, you are correct that a string of one-night stands will do little to achieve lasting fulfillment. Instead, try to build an emotional connection with your potential partner before you engage in sexual activity with her. That will have the biggest benefit for you in terms of an elevated emotional state, enhanced quality of life, and long-term fulfillment.

Bob: So should I add romance to the list of things I enjoy?

Carol: I find it quite interesting that this is the second time you mentioned romance when you started off talking only of sex. Whether you add that to your list is ultimately up to you. However, if you do choose to add it, you should understand that you need to have an emotional connection with your partner to achieve a lasting positive emotional impact. I also think the word "romance" is an appropriate one, as it implies both an emotional and physical connection.

Bob: Food for thought. Okay, I'll think that one over a bit more and decide if I want to include it. I do have another question regarding this list, though. I know it's about the things I enjoy, the things I want to do, but what about the things I have to do, what about chores? Do I need a separate list for those?

Carol: Good question. We all have chores we must do, such as paying bills, filing tax returns, and taking out the trash. Many people keep these tasks on a separate to-do list. However, there is no reason you cannot add those tasks to this list if you so choose. Just create two sub-categories, one called "Enjoyment" and one called "Chores." You can then add both types of activities to your list.

Bob: Okay, I think that works. I'll go ahead and build a list with those two headings.

Carol: One word of advice. When you build your list, try to achieve balance on it.

Bob: What does that mean?

Carol: It means balance out the activities you enjoy doing, with the activities that are chores. Try to make sure you have at least a 50/50 split. A 70/30 split is a bit better. You want to have at least as many activities on your list that you enjoy as ones that are chores. Otherwise, your list will turn into a mundane to-do list that will do nothing to elevate your spirits and bring you joy.

Bob: But what if I really have more chores than things I like to do?

Carol: I suspect that will not be the case, but if you do come up with a list that has more chores on it than things you enjoy, at least you will have a starting point to correct your out of balance situation. You can work to fix this, and over time, you will bring your list back into balance.

Bob: But why is balancing my list important?

Carol: Because a balanced list leads to a balanced life. Balance in life is extremely important. A life that is in balance is a life that is in equilibrium, a life that is stable, and a life that runs smoothly.

Bob: I'm not sure I understand.

Carol: Have you ever driven a car when the wheels were out of balance?

Bob: Yes, it was awful! The car shimmied, jittered, and rattled as I drove it down the highway.

Carol: That is because the out of balance tires affected the car's other systems, actually throwing other parts of the car out of balance. The same concept applies to your life. If something is out of balance in one area of your life, like a to-do list filled mainly with unpleasant or routine chores, it can throw other areas out of balance as well.

Bob: Okay, I get it, so I want to make sure my list of activities is properly balanced or it could negatively affect other areas of my life, is that correct?

Carol: Yes, you stated it correctly. And when you make your list, strive for balance, but don't be too hard on yourself if you do not achieve it on your first try. Over time, and with a concerted effort, you will eventually achieve balance on your list, and in your life.

Bob: And I assume you are going to show me how to use this list in our next session, correct?

Carol: Once again, you are correct.

Bob: Okay, on to the last item!

Carol: The last Spirit technique is – **Find some way to release your frustrations**.

Bob: Frustrations? But I thought the whole point of these techniques was to elevate my spirits and put me into a positive emotional state? If I do these other seven things, then won't I virtually eliminate all my frustrations?

Carol: In an ideal world, yes. In fact, these other seven techniques do serve to minimize your frustrations. We are all human beings, however, and we do experience negative emotions at times. Also, emotions are a form of energy, and negative energy is a natural part of the universe.

Bob: What do you mean?

Carol: Both positive and negative energy are required to achieve balance in the universe. One cannot exist without the other. For example, there are both positive and negative electrons in an atom. Batteries have both a positive and a negative charge. Magnets work because they contain both positive and negative forces that create a magnetic field. So you cannot entirely escape negative energy.

As humans, the key is to achieve balance, to keep both positive and negative energy in equilibrium within us. If these forces get out of balance, that is, become tilted too much towards the negative side, things such as frustration, fear, and anger might show up. Thoughts control this to some extent, but sometimes, you need a release. That is what this technique is all about.

Bob: So all that's great, but it's a bit too heavy on theory. How do I make practical use of this?

Carol: You want to find a way to release the negative energy from your body and your mind. This allows the positive energy to properly flow again, restoring your positive emotional state.

I have found that a great way to get rid of frustrations that rile me up is to do something physical, like work in my garden. For me, pulling weeds, cultivating soil, or raking up leaves that have fallen into the garden, gives me the physical activity I need to help me release pent up negative energy from my body. But gardening is only one example. There are a lot of things you can do to release negative energy from your body. Some people practice yoga, or go for a run, or even hit a punching bag.

Bob: Okay, I get your examples, but I'm not sure how getting rid of my frustrations helps me release negative energy.

Carol: Think about the last time you were really mad.

Bob: It was just last week. I had to deal with the phone company regarding my cable TV service. It took me hours; it was so frustrating!

Carol: What did you do after you hung up with the phone company?

Bob: I punched a wall.

Carol: Really?

Bob: No, of course not. But I felt like doing that.

Carol: Well, I can never advocate punching a wall with your bare hand. You could actually break it, making the problem even worse. However, you are on the right track.

Bob: What are you talking about?

Carol: Suppose instead of hitting a wall, you hit a punching bag several times. How would that feel?

Bob: I don't know, since I've never actually done that.

Carol: Okay, let's try something. I want you to close your eyes and replay in your mind the conversation with the phone company.

Bob: Okay, let me try ... Okay, I'm on the phone with the phone company, trying to get my cable TV service to work properly ... It's taking forever.

Carol: How do you feel now?

Bob: Frustrated!

Carol: Now I want you to visualize a punching bag. Visualize that it is right in front of you. Focus on its shape, its height, and its color ... Really try to see it.

Bob: Okay, I'm trying ... Wow! I can actually see it.

Carol: Okay, now I want you to punch it. Really punch it. If you want to physically swing at it, go ahead. There is nothing in front of you to get in your way, like a wall.

Bob: Okay, I'm swinging at it ... I'm actually hitting it!

Carol: Keep punching for at least 10 more seconds ... Now stop. How do you feel?

Bob: Strangely, I feel better. But how come?

Carol: When you relieved your frustration by hitting that imaginary punching bag, you released all of that negative energy from your body. That is why you feel better. Physical activity is one of the best ways to release frustration and negative energy, and it does not matter what that activity is. In my case it is gardening. In the exercise you just did, it was hitting a punching bag. But it could be anything – going for a walk, riding a bicycle, mowing the lawn, anything you can think of.

Bob: But I didn't actually do anything physical. I didn't really hit a punching bag. I only pretended to do that.

Carol: It does not matter whether you actually hit the punching bag; it is enough that you thought you did. Pretending to hit the punching bag had the same effect as if you had actually hit it. That is because the mind cannot distinguish between pretending to do something, and actually doing it.

Bob: Is that true?

Carol: Well, did you feel better after pretending to hit that punching bag?

Bob: Yes I did … Okay, now I get it.

Carol: Good, I am glad you are getting the concept. This is also the reason that athletes visualize performing their events. They are practicing their events in their minds. Visualization also works in areas besides athletics. As we just demonstrated, you can apply these concepts to much of your own life.

Bob: Fascinating! Can you tell me more about how and why visualization works?

Carol: Exploring this subject in more detail would get us a bit off track. However, there are several good books on visualization that you can purchase if you would like to read more about it. One that I like is titled *Creative Visualization,* but there are many other good books on the subject.[14]

Bob: That's good to know. Okay, so back to relieving frustrations. How can I make use of this technique?

Carol: As the final part of your homework, I want you to make a list of 10 physical activities that you can engage in when you become frustrated. They can be any safe activity that is physical. The key is to identify activities that you can do as soon as you become frustrated.

Bob: Why does it have to be something I can do right away?

Carol: Because you want to release that negative energy from your body as soon as you possibly can. Too much negative energy is not good for you.

Bob: Yes, I see that now. Okay, I'll add this to my list of things to work on for next week.

Carol: Well, we have covered a lot of ground, and you should feel good about your accomplishments.

Bob: I do.

Carol: Good, I do as well. I will see you next Tuesday at 3 PM then?

Bob: Already looking forward to it. Have a good evening, Carol, and thanks.

Carol: You're welcome, Bob. You have a nice evening as well, and a good week.

———— ⊗ ————

Bob gets up and leaves the room. Carol breathes a sigh of relief. She was initially stunned at the start of the session by Bob's violent resistance. Fortunately, she has been doing this a long time and has seen worse reactions than Bob's, so she was prepared for the encounter. She got him through the session today, however, and it appeared to end well – Bob took his homework assignments and promised to complete them by their next meeting.

However, Carol has an uneasy feeling. She's not sure Bob has completely bought in yet. She's sensing strong resistance, but she's not sure where it's coming from. After thinking about it, Carol decides that Bob's resistance will break down naturally during the course of their sessions ... she hopes.

Bob was her last appointment for the day, so Carol decides to head out while the sun is still shining so she can watch the sunset, something that brings her great pleasure.

———⚬———

Bob is muttering to himself on his drive home. "I shouldn't have been so negative at the start of the session today. I kind of see the value in Carol's techniques, but I have a hard time believing they will really help me. I just don't know if there's any hope for me."

Bob promises himself he will try to do Carol's homework assignments as best he can. With that, he turns on the car radio and tunes it to his favorite station, a political talk station.

As Bob listens to the radio host and callers debate the political topics of the day, he feels his blood pressure starting to rise. He continues to drive home, unaware of the magnificent sunset occurring right before his eyes.

CHAPTER 4

Spirit: Part II

It has been one week since Carol's last session with Bob, and she's anxious to see his homework assignments. She's also excited for today, as this is the session where patients really begin to customize their journey and choose their own path. This is the session where patients start to realize that they do, in fact, have the power of choice.

If everything has gone according to plan, Bob will have already started to realize this while doing his homework assignments. Carol cannot wait to see what Bob has discovered; she's almost giddy with anticipation.

———◉———

Bob sits quietly in the waiting room, nervous about his upcoming session with Carol. Several times during the week, he'd thought about calling to cancel this appointment, and all his appointments for the coming weeks. But he didn't. Something inside him told him this was an important appointment, and that he might learn something about himself that would finally allow him to conquer his inner doom.

It's Tuesday at 2:58 PM. As the hour approaches, Bob's heart begins to beat a bit faster, and he starts to perspire slightly. Just then, Carol walks out to greet him. Bob tentatively rises from his chair with a forced half-grin, and allows Carol to usher him into her office.

——————⊛——————

Carol: Hello Bob, how are you today?

Bob: Um … I'm okay.

Carol: Just okay? So, I have been anxiously waiting all week; tell me how your homework assignments went.

Bob: Well … I didn't get to them, actually.

Carol: I see. Would you tell me why?

Bob: Well, I went home, and was eager to start. I sat down, but drew a blank; I had no idea what to write. So I decided I needed to clear my head and relax. I thought that would get my mind working.

Carol: That sounds like a good thought.

Bob: Yeah, well … I went to the bar and had a couple of drinks, and that got me to thinking.

Carol: What did you think about?

Bob: I thought about how all your homework assignments were really going to be a lot of work, and I wondered if they were actually going to help me. I mean, I'm sure your techniques have worked for other patients, but there's no guarantee they will help me! Then I remembered something I almost forgot. I remembered that our path in life is predetermined, no matter how hard we pretend it's not. No matter how hard we try, we can't escape our fate. I KNOW we have no choice. We're doomed to follow our predetermined path, whatever it is. That's what I know; the rest of this is all bullshit!

Carol: Clearly, you have thought a lot about this.

Bob: Yes, and what's more, as I was sitting at the bar having a few drinks, I noticed I started to become more relaxed, I noticed my stress levels went down, and I noticed my mood got better. In short, I noticed I started to enjoy myself! So that's what I did for fun this past week, I went to the bar every night for a few drinks. And you know what? It worked! So it looks like I can use that to improve my spirits instead of going through all this therapy stuff.

Carol: I understand, and while it is true that going to the bar and consuming alcohol each night has worked to lift your spirits, the effect is only going to be temporary. During our first session, you mentioned that your daily, or nightly, routine was sitting around drinking, eating, and watching TV. Do you remember how you felt in my office that day? You were somewhat exasperated, and you instinctively knew that behavior could not go on forever.

Bob: Yeah, so what's your point?

Carol: Before long, you will need to consume more alcohol to achieve the same effect that a drink or two once had. Eventually, instead of lifting your spirits, the alcohol will have the opposite effect.

Bob: What do you mean by "the opposite effect"?

Carol: Did you ever drink too much? Perhaps when you were out with friends, or at a Christmas party?

Bob: I can remember several times I did that, actually.

Carol: Do you remember how you felt the next morning?

Bob: Well, when I was a young man, excess alcohol had no effect on me. I was up all the earlier the next morning. As I grew older, though, I noticed I started getting hangovers the next day. I generally felt miserable, and didn't want to do much of anything except sit around and watch TV all day.

Carol: Exactly. As we get older, our bodies lose the ability to metabolize alcohol efficiently. What's more, prolonged excess consumption of alcohol can have serious impacts on the human body, and can cause things such as liver or heart disease.[15]

Bob: I know all that, but I went to the bar all last week, and I felt fine ... I mean ... I've learned my lesson, and I can handle it now ... I mean ... Oh, damnit! Okay, I see what you mean. So what are you saying, that I can never have another drink for as long as I live?

Carol: No, of course not. In fact, I have wine once in a while myself. Everything in moderation. We will discuss that in more detail when we have our session on Body.

Bob: Okay, I get it. Going to the bar isn't the answer. So what is?

Carol: Well, instead of relying on external stimulants, a better approach is to inspire happiness, health, and fulfillment from within, which is the point of the homework assignments I gave you last week.

Bob: I guess you're right. I should do the assignments. After all, I'm the one who came to you for help. The thing is, I don't know where to start, and I'm afraid I'll just slip back into my old ways if I get stuck again.

Carol: In that case, let's use our session today to complete these exercises. I will help you with each one.

Bob: Okay. I'd appreciate that. Where do we begin?

Carol: With the first assignment for the first technique – **Be thankful for what you have**. I want you to list out at least 10 things you are thankful for. Let's do that right now.

To the Reader:

Can you help Bob complete this list? Go to Appendix A and find the section titled **"Be thankful for what you have."** Complete this list before reading on.

Bob: Okay, I think I have a good list here. Now how do I use it?

Carol: Review this list daily. Place it somewhere you can see it, like on your bathroom mirror, or on a wall next to your dresser – anywhere you are sure to see it each day. Then, each time you see this list, review it and really think about how thankful you are for everything you have in your life. Doing this will help you realize how much you have in your life that is positive, and how much you truly have to be thankful for – which will lift your spirits and put you into a positive emotional state.

Bob: But that seems like a lot of work. Do I really have to do this daily?

Carol: It is good to do this daily, as it helps ingrain the habit. At first, any new habit seems like a lot of work because it is something different, something new. That is precisely why I suggest putting the list up where you will naturally see it each day. You will not have to worry about remembering to do this exercise; seeing this list will automatically remind you to do it.

Bob: Got it. And it's not like I have a full schedule every day, so I guess I can do this. Okay, what's next?

Carol: The next assignment was related to the second technique – **Surround yourself with family.** I want you to make a list of your family members. This list can include either blood relatives, adopted family, or both. Next to the name of each family member, write the current state of your relationship with them. For example, is your relationship with them good, or is it strained? How close do you currently feel to them, very close or very distant? How do you feel emotionally when you think of them? Do you feel happy, or angry, or sad?

If you are not on good terms with a particular family member, it will also help to write down what caused the relationship to become strained. This will give you a perspective that might prove helpful when you begin to repair the relationship. Go ahead and take a few minutes and do that now.

To the Reader:

Can you help Bob complete this assignment? Go to Appendix A and find the section titled **"Surround yourself with family."** Complete the relevant columns of this table before reading on.

Bob: Okay, done with homework assignment number two. So how do I use this list?

Carol: In two ways. First, make time to keep in touch with the family members on your list that you have good relationships with. You may want to contact them daily, weekly, or monthly, depending on how close you are. How often you contact them is up to you. I would say, however, that you want to make sure to contact each family member you have a good relationship with at least once a month. That way, you will be sure not to lose touch with them.

It can also be useful to schedule a specific time on your calendar to call each family member. You can make it a recurring appointment if you want to. That way, your calendar will serve as a "keep in touch" reminder for you.

Bob: Makes sense. What's the second way?

Carol: The second way pertains to family members you have strained relations with. These negative relationships can actually cause you tension, stress, and anxiety every time you think of, or talk to, any of these people.

Bob: Okay, but what can I do about it?

Carol: You will want to remove this negativity from your life. The more you can minimize relationship negativity, such as drama and tension, the happier you will be. If these relationships are important to you, say a relationship with your mother that is currently strained, then you will want to work to improve it. If, on the other hand, the relationship is not one that you care about, say one with a distant cousin, then you may want to just leave it alone, or even cut that person out of your life. How you specifically choose to deal with each one of these strained relationships is entirely up to you. Again, it is all about choice, and the choice is ultimately yours to make.

Bob: Cut family members out of my life? That sounds a bit harsh!

Carol: It may seem that way right now, but remember, this is YOUR happiness, health, and fulfillment we are talking about, and relationships are a two-way street. If the other person is not contributing to your joy and contentment, if you tense up or experience dread every time you talk to them, then the relationship is ultimately doing you more harm than good. You will either need to repair or eliminate that relationship. In the end, this will be better for everyone.

Bob: You know, as you were saying that, it got me to thinking. My kids and I really haven't spoken since they graduated college and moved away.

Carol: Would you tell me a bit more about that?

Bob: Well, the last time I saw my kids, it didn't end well. Remember I told you that they acted like entitled spoiled brats? Well, that continued until they graduated college. In fact, I refused to let them move back home after school. I wanted them to learn what it was like to be on their own.

Carol: You threw them out?

Bob: It's called tough love! Anyway, my kids and I haven't really spoken since. I would like to try and rebuild my relationship with them, but where do I start? I mean, what if they reject me?

Carol: Start with an in-person conversation, or even a phone call. Be open with them. Tell them they are important to you, and that you want to work on improving your relationship with them. If they care about you, then they should respond positively.

Bob: But what if they don't? What if they don't want to make things better?

Carol: Well, wouldn't you rather know that now instead of spending years driving yourself crazy over how to repair a relationship that is beyond hope?

Bob: I see your point. The more negativity I can eliminate, especially at this stage in my life, the better.

Carol: Exactly.

Bob: Okay, what's next?

Carol: The next assignment was related to the third technique –

Have close friends. To start with, review the list of family members you compiled as part of the second technique – **Surround yourself with family** – and add the names of your close friends. Now, for each person on your list, I want you to mark whether they are an Eeyore. Take a few minutes and do this now.

To the Reader:

Can you help Bob complete this assignment? Go to Appendix A and find the section titled **"Have close friends."** Update the relevant columns of this table before reading on.

Bob: Okay, I'm done updating my list. I think I know how to use it based on what we've already talked about, except how do I use this new Eeyore column?

Carol: This new column identifies the Eeyores in your life, and you want to use it to help you avoid them at all costs.

Bob: Even my close friends?

Carol: Especially your close friends. Eeyores carry negative energy with them wherever they go. They always have a dark cloud hanging over their heads. If you stand too close to them, then you will also be covered by their dark cloud. This will drain your energy and negatively affect your mood, thus putting you into a negative emotional state.

Bob: So just associating with negative people will drain my energy? I find that hard to believe.

Carol: It's true. Eeyores crave attention and sympathy; they feed off it. Eeyores consume other people's positive energy. In return, they give back negative energy, which has a damaging effect on a person's emotional state. The Eeyore closely resembles the "Victim" in the Karpman Drama Triangle.[16] Victims have a "poor me" disposition, and they are masters at manipulating you into pitying them. They are always seeking someone to come in and "save the day." But no matter how much energy and attention you give them, they will always have another reason for you to feel sorry for them, and they will eventually wind up drawing you into their den of misery.

Bob: Now that you put it that way, I understand. But cutting off my friends seems cold.

Carol: Remember, your goal is to achieve happiness, health, and fulfillment. To do this, you need to surround yourself with people, events, and things that bring you joy, and distance yourself from the people, events, and things that bring you misery.

Bob: Okay, I get your point. I'll minimize the amount of time I spend with my close friends who are Eeyores.

Carol: It's not just your close friends; Eeyores are everywhere. Even a distant acquaintance can drain your energy if you hang around them long enough. Be on the lookout for Eeyores wherever they are and avoid them at all costs.

Bob: This topic is fascinating. Can you tell me more about this "Drama Triangle" thing?

Carol: That would actually take us off course, but you are right, it is a fascinating subject. If you are interested in learning more about it, there are several books written about the Drama Triangle that you can read. There is even one written by the creator of the Drama Triangle, Dr. Stephen Karpman. The book is called *A Game Free Life.*[17]

Bob: Interesting, maybe I'll check it out. Okay, what's next?

Carol: So, moving on, the next assignment was related to the fourth technique – **Be happy for others' good fortune.** Continuing from the last exercise, take the list of family and friends you started and build on it. For each person on your list, I want you to think of something good that has happened to them and write that next to their name. Go ahead and do that now.

To the Reader:

Can you help Bob complete this assignment? Go to Appendix A and find the section titled **"Be happy for others' good fortune."** Update this table before reading on.

Bob: Okay, I'm done with this assignment. Same question, how do I use it?

Carol: Call each person on your list and express your happiness for them and their good fortune. Gratitude for someone else will automatically bring you happiness. This is in accordance with the Law of Compensation,[18] which states that you will be justly compensated for what you give, but you must give it first. Give gratitude, get thanks, and receive happiness.

Bob: I see.

Carol: This technique also works for repairing damaged relationships. If something good has happened to a person you are currently estranged from, call them up and express your happiness for their good fortune. They will appreciate your thoughtfulness, and this will be an important first step towards rebuilding your relationship with them.

Bob: But what if I can't think of anything good that has happened to one of my friends, or to my strained relations, particularly the ones I haven't kept in touch with?

Carol: Call them anyway. Most people will have something good happen to them sooner or later, and even if it is a small thing, they will be eager to share it with someone they are close to. Keep the conversation going, and they will eventually share some good news with you. Just be sure to express your happiness for them when they do.

Bob: Okay. Kind of feels like my to-do list is starting to grow, but at least we're making good progress with these assignments. What's next?

Carol: The next assignment was related to the fifth technique – **Look at the beauty of nature around you.** I want you to write down at least 10 things that you find beautiful in nature. You already started this list for me in our last session when you gave me the things you enjoy about fall: the changing of the leaves, the apple-picking, and the harvest dinners. Take a few minutes and do this now.

To the Reader:

Can you help Bob complete this assignment? Go to Appendix A and find the section titled **"Look at the beauty of nature around you."** Complete this list before reading on.

Bob: Okay, I've completed the list. So how do I use it?

Carol: First, I want you to place this list where you can see it. You can put it up anywhere you pass frequently. Like your other list, you may want to place this one on your bathroom mirror, or next to your dresser. You may even want to put it up on your refrigerator.

Bob: Okay, once I have the list up, then what?

Carol: Review it on a daily basis. Then, each day, go out into the world and actually observe, or physically experience, one of the things in nature you find beautiful. For instance, if it is the fall season, and you enjoy watching the leaves changing colors, take a walk and actually observe them with your own eyes. Or if you enjoy fresh vegetables, go to a farmer's market, or even the produce section of your local grocery store, and observe nature's bounty. If you like the mountains or the rolling hills, go for a drive in the countryside. While you are there, stop your car, get out, look around you, and experience the environment.

Bob: I see, so just take time to look at the things in nature I find beautiful, right?

Carol: Do not just look at them, EXPERIENCE them with as many of your senses as possible. See the colors, smell the fragrant air, listen to the rustling leaves or the birds twittering in the trees. Go to a farm stand and buy a crisp apple and bite into it. Concentrate on its taste, texture, and aroma. Is it sweet or tart? Is it juicy? Smell it. Feel the smooth skin. This is how you EXPERIENCE something. Then, focus on how this makes you feel. Feel the joy the experience brings you. This will elevate your spirits and put you into a positive emotional state.

Bob: Okay, I get it, but how is this different from the first technique? You know, the one where I am thankful for what I have?

Carol: The things you have on your list for the first technique can be either tangible or intangible; in actual existence physically, or in existence only as an event, thought, or personality trait. The items on this list are all in physical existence, meaning you can actually experience them with your five senses.

Bob: But why is that important?

Carol: Because we are all driven by our senses. It is easier for us to appreciate and believe what is in physical existence than it is for us to appreciate and believe what is not.

Bob: I'm still not sure I get it.

Carol: The easier it is for you to experience joy, the better. And things that physically exist are easier for you to appreciate and experience. Positive emotions, and a positive emotional state, follow as a matter of course.

Bob: Okay, I understand, in theory at least. But isn't this the same as relying on external things for happiness?

Carol: As human beings, we have been given five senses so we can experience the environment. We were not meant to live in a vacuum; in fact, it is unhealthy for us to do so. Think of a person who is bed-ridden, or lives their life in total isolation, either unable or unwilling to go out and interact with the world. The quality of life for most of these people is usually substandard. Engaging with the natural environment is different from relying on external stimulation for happiness.

Bob: How so?

Carol: The external activities we typically engage in – such as taking a cruise or going on vacation – are designed to help us escape our lives, at least temporarily, which is very different from engaging with the natural environment.

Bob: Huh … I never thought about it that way.

Carol: Also, our problems are still there waiting for us when we come back from whatever means we use to achieve our temporary escape. And, as we get older and become less mobile, we slowly lose our ability to escape our lives – escape our personal environments.

Bob: That sounds depressing.

Carol: While aging is a fact of life, there is no reason it has to be unpleasant. It is just a matter of how you choose to experience *your* environment. This exercise, and every other exercise I have given you, has to do with changing how you choose to respond to your environment; getting you to open your eyes and see all the good things you already have in your life that you can feel happy about.

Also, the techniques I am teaching you will always be with you. No matter how old you get, you can always use them to elevate your spirits and put yourself into a positive emotional state. So even if you cannot change your environment, you CAN change the way you choose to experience it.

Bob: Alright, I see your points. I'll make sure to add this to my daily routine. What's next?

Carol: The next assignment was related to the sixth technique – **Do something for someone else.** I want you to make a list of at least 10 things you have done for someone else. These things could either be in the recent or distant past. Next to each item, write down how that good deed made you feel, and how you were compensated for it. Remember, your compensation does not necessarily come from the person you did the good deed for, nor does it necessarily immediately follow the good deed. Compensation can come days, months, or even years afterward.

If you do not recognize how you were compensated for a specific action, just leave a blank next to it. However, for each action on your list, do write down how it made you feel. That part is important. Take a moment and do this now.

To the Reader:

Can you help Bob complete this assignment? Go to Appendix A and find the section titled **"Do something for someone else."** Complete this table before reading on.

Bob: Okay, I'm done with this list, so how do I use it?

Carol: Just as you are going to do with your other lists, hang this one up in a place you will pass frequently, like your bathroom mirror or your refrigerator. Each morning when you see this list, review each item, think about the good deed you did, the person you did it for, and how it made you feel. Then close your eyes for a few minutes and experience the emotions those good deeds gave you. This will elevate your mood, and put you into a positive emotional state.

Bob: Okay, I will add this to my routine. Looks like my daily activities are really starting to pile up. This seems like a lot of work to do each day. I had no idea this was going to be that much of a chore!

Carol: Any new routine will seem like a lot of effort at first. Remember, these are new habits you are forming, and any new habit takes effort and practice before it becomes ingrained. How you view these exercises also affects how burdensome they feel to you. You can either view them as a daily chore, which is a heavy burden, or you can view them as something that will help you reach your life goals, which is not a burden at all.

Bob: Still seems like a lot of work to do each day.

Carol: I understand, and I don't want you to feel overwhelmed. Otherwise, you may not do *any* of these exercises.

Bob: Right, and I want to do them. I want to change my life; it just seems like so much work.

Carol: Right now, it feels that way, but soon this new routine will become automatic. And as these exercises begin to have a positive effect, you will want to keep doing them, perhaps even more often.

Bob: Seems hard to believe.

Carol: At the start of their journeys, many of my former patients felt the same way you do right now. Any new activity you engage in feels difficult and awkward at first. Think about when you first learned to drive a car. Do you remember what that was like?

Bob: Yeah, it was frustrating. There were so many things I needed to keep in my head, and all at the same time. I thought I'd never learn.

Carol: And today?

Bob: Now I hardly think about it; it's automatic. I just get in the car and go.

Carol: The same principles apply here. However, to make this less overwhelming for you, let's space these exercises out a bit.

Bob: Sounds good, but how?

Carol: Start by blocking out a limited amount of time each day to work on these exercises. Let's begin with 15 minutes a day. The first day, spend those 15 minutes working on only one, maybe two, exercises. The next day, spend those 15 minutes working on a different exercise or two. That way, you will be able to complete all your exercises within a week's time.

Bob: That sounds a bit more manageable.

Carol: Also, make sure to use your calendar to schedule different exercises each day; do not do the same ones daily. It is like working out at the gym. You may work out daily, but you do not want to work the same muscle groups each day. That would just lead to fatigue and boredom, which is something you are trying to avoid.

Bob: Okay, I'll make use of a calendar, spread these exercises out, and do different ones each day. What's next?

Carol: The next assignment was related to the seventh technique – **Do the things you enjoy doing.** Make a list of at least 10 things you enjoy doing. You can put anything on this list, whether you have done it yet or not. You might include only enjoyable things you have done in the past, but you can also include things you have not done yet, but might enjoy doing in the future.

If you want to add routine chores to your list, create two sub-categories, one called "Enjoyment" and one called "Chores." You can then add both types of activities to the same list. If you build your list this way, try to balance the activities you enjoy doing with the activities that are chores. Try to make sure you have at least a 50/50 split. A 70/30 split is better.

Remember, you want to have at least as many activities on your list that you enjoy as ones that are chores. Otherwise your list will turn into a mundane to-do list that will do nothing to elevate your spirits and bring you joy.

Take a few minutes and complete this list now.

To the Reader:

Can you help Bob complete this assignment? Go to Appendix A and find the section titled **"Do the things you enjoy doing."** Complete this table before reading on.

Bob: Okay, I'm done with this list. Should I use it the same way as the other lists?

Carol: You will use this list to remind yourself of the things that you enjoy. Each day, make sure you schedule yourself for at least one enjoyable activity from this list; more than one would be better, but make sure you schedule at least one. That way, you will always have something fun to look forward to every day.

Bob: That's it? Seems too simple.

Carol: It is fairly simple; however, there are some things to keep in mind. Just as you did when you made your list, make sure that you achieve balance in your daily activities. As we discussed, balance is important in all aspects of life. You want to eventually get into the habit of spending at least half of your day doing the things you enjoy doing.

Ideally, you would spend your whole day doing only the things you enjoy doing, but this may be a bit unrealistic, so try to achieve at least a 50/50 split in your daily activities; striving for a 70/30 split would be even better.

Bob: Okay, I'll try. Any other advice on how to use this list?

Carol: Yes. Make sure you achieve balance with the things you enjoy doing. For instance, if you like watching TV, or movies, make sure you do not spend your entire day doing only that. And please, don't make this the ONLY activity you do day after day; that would actually have the opposite effect and make you unhappy in the long run.

Bob: So do you have any suggestions on how I should achieve this balance?

Carol: Spread your activities around. If you enjoy watching TV, do that for an hour or two, then get out and do something else. Go out to lunch, or go play cards with friends. Also, try to balance physical versus sedentary activities. Start with a 50/50 split. If you spend an hour or two watching TV, then spend the next hour or two doing something physical – like taking a walk, exercising, or playing nine holes of golf.

Bob: That actually sounds good. I'll make sure to balance my daily activities. What's next?

Carol: The next assignment was related to the eighth technique
– **Find some way to release your frustrations.** Make a list of 10
physical activities you can engage in when you become frustrated. They can be any safe activity that is physical. The key is to
identify activities you can do as soon as you become frustrated.
For this list, let me give you a couple of tips before you begin.

It goes without saying, but make sure the activities you choose
are legal and safe. Shooting a gun is fine, but make sure you do it
at an authorized shooting range, not out in public, and shoot at
something that is legal to shoot at, like paper targets. Also, make
sure you engage in frustration releasing behavior that is not destructive. For instance, if you find yourself breaking plates and
glasses against a wall or worse, throwing them at someone, your
frustration has turned into destructive behavior. Destructive activities are not ones that you want to include on your list.

Bob: Of course! I'd never do something that would hurt anyone.
So I need to list things that are physical, but not destructive to me
or someone else.

Carol: Correct, and make sure that includes you. By that I mean,
avoid things that are dangerous to your health and well-being.
For example, if you want to punch something, choose to hit a
pillow or a punching bag, not a wall.

Bob: Okay, I'll keep all that in mind as I make up my list.

Carol: Good. So now you can proceed. Take a few minutes and list out these activities now.

To the Reader:

Can you help Bob complete this assignment? Go to Appendix A and find the section titled **"Find some way to release your frustrations."** Complete this list before reading on.

Bob: Okay, I've completed this list. Same question as before, how do I use it?

Carol: Take this list and put it in your wallet. Take it with you wherever you go. When you become frustrated, look at the list, and try to identify an activity you can do right away to release your frustrations.

Remember, frustration carries negative energy. Once it takes hold of you, everything that follows generally takes on a negative aspect. Your outlook will be negatively affected, and you will wind up making poor decisions as a result, which will only make things worse for you. So you will want to release this negative energy from your body before it ruins your day.

Bob: So I should look to do one of these things the minute I become frustrated. Correct?

Carol: Yes, within reason. For example, if screaming at the top of your lungs is one of the activities on your list, do not stand in the middle of a waiting room full of people at your doctor's office and scream. Wait to scream until you are alone, perhaps within the confines of your car.

Bob: Understood. Good advice.

Carol: Well, we had a long but very productive day today. You should feel proud of what you have accomplished.

Bob: I do. Thanks for helping me through these assignments. One more question. When do I begin using these lists?

Carol: You can begin using them immediately. Take the list of things you can do to release your frustrations and put it into your wallet right now. Start using that list the very next time you become frustrated. Go home tonight and put up the other lists where you can see them. Then either tonight or tomorrow morning, take a look at them and start to do the exercises. Also, immediately add the exercises to your daily calendar. You want to start forming these new habits as quickly as possible – while you have the momentum and enthusiasm from this session.

Bob: Okay, I'll do that. Thanks for the advice. See you same time next week?

Carol: Absolutely. I am looking forward to it.

Bob: Okay, thanks again for today, and have a good evening.

Carol: You too, Bob.

———⊛———

Carol doesn't know whether to celebrate or collapse. The session today was another successful one, and she was able to help Bob complete the assignments that will ultimately help him realize his goals. Still, it was exhausting, and she feels a bit tired. Fortunately, this was her last appointment for the day. She decides to leave early, watch another sunset, marvel at nature's wonders, have an early dinner, and turn in for the evening.

———⊛———

Bob is excited as he drives home.

Finally, it looks like I've found someone who can actually help me! he thinks.

As soon as he gets home, he eagerly puts up the lists on his bathroom mirror and begins scheduling out his daily exercises. Things are off to a good start, and Bob anxiously anticipates the new insights he will get in his next few sessions with Carol.

Bob continues working on his schedule. He is determined to get all his new exercises scheduled before he turns in for the evening.

CHAPTER 5

Mind

Carol sits quietly in her office. It's 2:55 PM on Tuesday afternoon; five minutes before her next session with Bob. Carol is looking forward to today's session. This is the session where she will teach Bob about MIND, and the major part it plays in happiness, health, and fulfillment.

This is also a major part of her "secret sauce," as she knows, through her years of experience as a medical practitioner, that the medical profession has largely ignored the importance of the mind in the practice of patient care, preferring to focus almost exclusively on the human body. While Carol knows that care of the human body is vitally important to happiness, health, and fulfillment, she knows it is only one part of the equation.

It's 2:59 PM, and Carol gets up from her chair and walks out to the waiting room to greet Bob. An eternal optimist, Carol is hopeful that Bob will be less resistant at the start of this session than he was at the start of the last two. She opens the door and sees Bob in the waiting room. He rises from his chair and walks into Carol's office, ready to begin round three.

———————— ◎ ————————

Carol: Hello Bob, how are you today?

Bob: Fine Carol, and you?

Carol: I am well, thank you. Today, we are going to discuss Mind, which is the second piece of ground we will be covering during our journey through Mind, Body, and Spirit.

Bob: Okay, tell me about Mind.

Carol: Mind plays a vital part in the quest for happiness, health, and fulfillment. Studies have shown that mental attitude can actually impact a person's emotional and physical states – either positively or negatively.[19]

Bob: Wait, you just mentioned all three areas – Mind, Body, and Spirit. I thought we were just talking about Mind?

Carol: Remember that all three areas are interrelated, so it is impossible to talk about one area without talking about how it affects the other two.

Bob: Okay, understood. So tell me more about Mind.

Carol: There are nine key things that help my patients achieve a healthy mindset and a positive mental attitude. I will list them out for you, then we can discuss each one in more detail.

1. Keep informed
2. Keep up your physical appearance
3. Live your life regardless of your age
4. Live in the present
5. Push yourself to participate
6. Do it now
7. Keep your mind fit
8. Keep in touch with time
9. Continue to learn

Bob: Once again, I see a list of techniques, and it looks like there are going to be exercises ... This seems like a hell of a lot of work to go through. What if none of this stuff works?

Carol: Well, how did the Spirit exercises go? Did they work to lift your spirits?

Bob: At first, then not so much.

Carol: I see. Tell me about that.

Bob: Well, I went home last week all excited; I couldn't wait to get started. I set up everything as soon as I got home, and did my exercises first thing the next morning. Surprisingly, I felt better almost immediately. I got excited that this stuff was actually working.

Carol: That sounds positive. So what happened after that?

Bob: I flipped on the TV, which is preset to my favorite cable news channel.

Carol: Do you watch that channel often?

Bob: All the time. In fact, it's the only channel I have on when I'm at home. I watch it all day. It gives me something to do.

Carol: I see. Tell me what happened as you watched that channel.

Bob: It actually started to depress me. Seems like there's so much misery and strife in the world. War, hunger, drought, natural disasters … It's everywhere, and it seems to be happening all day, every day.

Carol: And what did that make you think about?

Bob: I got to thinking that no matter what we do, we have no choice, no control. I see it on the TV and in the news each day. All the disaster and suffering in the world … Seems like it just happens automatically, and there's nothing anyone can do to stop it. It's so depressing!

Carol: And what did you do after you watched TV?

Bob: Nothing! I felt so depressed after watching the news, I really didn't feel like doing anything. I actually felt tired, like I needed a nap or something.

Carol: What about the next day?

Bob: Same thing. I did the exercises, started to feel good, then turned on the cable news, watched for a bit, then became depressed at all the strife and misery going on.

Carol: And the next day?

Bob: Just turned on the news. I decided doing the exercises is pointless. The positive effects just get wiped out as soon as daily life starts to intervene, and I can't prevent life from intervening. I have no control over that.

Carol: While it is true that you cannot prevent bad things from happening in the world, you can control how much of that you let into your life, and how you allow it to affect your mood.

Bob: What do you mean?

Carol: Tell me a little bit about what you saw on the news this morning? What natural disasters took place?

Bob: I saw that there was an earthquake in Nepal, a fire in the Amazon rainforest, and a typhoon in Japan … They said all of this was caused by global warming.

Carol: Okay, do you live in any of these areas of the world, and are you personally affected by any of these particular recent disasters?

Bob: Well, no.

Carol: And yet you allow them to affect your mood. You allow them to take over your life and affect how you feel and act, even though these disasters do not touch your life. What would you do if you did not know about these disasters? What would you do if you had no idea these things were occurring in the world? How would they affect you?

Bob: I don't know ... They wouldn't, I guess.

Carol: Exactly.

Bob: What's your point?

Carol: My point is that you do have control over what you let into your life and into your environment.

Bob: What do you mean by that? My environment is the world I live in. How can I control that?

Carol: Environment is more than just the physical aspects of the world. But let's say, for the moment, that environment just represents the physical world. The world is a big place. There is a global environment – the planet we live on, and a local environment – the country, state, city, neighborhood, or even the street we live on.

Bob: I'm not sure I'm following you.

Carol: The fact that something is happening in another part of the world does not typically affect *your* specific environment, which is usually limited to the few miles surrounding your home and the places you frequent.

Bob: Okay, but that doesn't negate the fact something bad is happening in another part of the world.

Carol: True. However, you can choose whether to let that event into your environment.

Bob: What do you mean by that?

Carol: Environment is more than just a geographic spot on the map, it is literally everything that you come into contact with – people, places, events, and thoughts. Moreover, you have control over what you let into your personal environment.

Bob: But how can I control what I let into my personal environment?

Carol: You can do that by choosing your thoughts carefully, and by being selective of who you let into your life. Most of the time, the thoughts and people we let into our lives are negative.

When we let negative events into our lives, it has an unavoidable negative impact on us, and affects both our emotional and mental states.

Let's go back to the cable news you watched yesterday morning. It clearly affected your mood in a negative way. Yet, you did not have to turn on the TV, or watch the news endlessly. You had almost complete control over what you let into your life yesterday. In fact, you have almost complete control over what you let into your life *every day.*

This leads me to the first Mind technique – **Keep informed.**

Bob: What does that mean?

Carol: You want to keep your mind active. Your brain is similar to a muscle. Without use, it can atrophy over time. Simply put, you either use it or lose it. Keeping informed – keeping up to date with current events – provides you with a way to use your mind on a daily basis, which keeps it active and healthy.

Bob: I don't see the difference between what you're saying and what I do each day. You just got done telling me how bad it is for me to let all of this negative stuff into my environment, and into my mind, by watching the cable news, and now you're telling me to keep informed on a daily basis?

Carol: There is a difference between keeping informed and inundating yourself with negative information. Constantly watching cable TV news, which is rarely positive, is akin to inundating yourself with negative information. And there are other ways to keep informed.

Bob: Okay, well what are some of these other ways?

Carol: You could read a newspaper, listen to news radio for 20 minutes each morning, or watch a local TV news show, which typically lasts only 30 minutes.

Bob: What's the difference where and how I get my news? Can't I just continue to watch my favorite cable news channel to keep informed?

Carol: You can, and by all means continue to do so if you want. Just do not watch it in a constant stream, that just inundates you with too much negative information too quickly.

Bob: What do you mean?

Carol: A cable TV news show is really just a highly compressed version of a newspaper. When you watch these types of shows, you are continually bombarded with highly concentrated news stories and graphic images designed to "inform" you almost instantaneously. Newspapers are designed to get you to spend more time with them, so any negative information in them is a bit more spread out. You do not get as much negative news as quickly when you read a newspaper.

Bob: Okay, that makes sense, I think.

Carol: And typical cable TV news shows just repeat the same news stories throughout the day. So not only are you getting negative news the first thing in the morning, but it is also being reinforced in your mind throughout the day. Even if you have the cable news on while you are doing other things and are not actually sitting in front of the TV, that negativity is continuing to flow to you, as if through a subliminal energy field.

Bob: I see.

Carol: Cable news programming is more about what will entertain, rather than inform, and you simply do not need this type of information to live your daily life.

A long time ago, I was just like you. I loved watching cable news shows. I felt that they kept me well informed. One day, I was watching a news segment about an important public policy issue, something on healthcare I think it was. I was very interested to learn about the particulars of this policy, the benefits as well as the drawbacks. The news anchor had two guest commentators on the show, each with opposing points of view. That should have been sufficient for the key issues to be debated out.

Bob: I would think so. So what happened?

Carol: Well, the two commentators spent their time insulting each other, and either ridiculing the other's policy or defending their own. When the 90 seconds of allotted air time was up, the anchor cut each of them off and thanked them for providing the public with great insight.

Bob: Sounds like you didn't learn anything.

Carol: That's the point. That news program provided no real news, no real information, it just provided conflict and drama. In fact, the only thing I got from that segment was angry. From that day forward, I have not watched a cable TV news program. I can live quite well without it, and I am much happier for it.

Bob: Okay, I get it. Too much negative news is bad for my mental attitude. So what other news formats would you suggest?

Carol: I suggest reading the first two columns on the front page of the *Wall Street Journal*. Not only do they have a nice summary of each day's US and global economic issues, but they also reference the full articles in the paper if you want to read more about a particular topic. You can also get everything you need from reading the first section of your daily local newspaper.

If you do not want to take that much time, there are several good news aggregator websites you can use to create a customized daily news digest. Again, it is all about choice, and today, you have more choices than ever about how to stay informed.

Bob: Okay, so if I've got this straight, I should exercise my mind by keeping informed on a daily basis, but I shouldn't focus too much on the negative things going on in the world because that will bring me down and do me more harm than good. Is that a good way of saying it?

Carol: Excellent summary.

Bob: Thanks, I think I'm finally getting the hang of this Mind stuff. So what's next?

Carol: **Keep up your physical appearance.**

Bob: Why is that important? I thought all of this was about the "inner self"? Not caring what the outside world thinks of me, but instead what I think of myself.

Carol: It is, and keeping up your physical appearance figures prominently in how you feel about yourself.

Bob: How?

Carol: Once again, it is about the environment we put ourselves into. Environment tends to affect how we feel about ourselves, both positively and negatively. And your body is a major part of your environment. Just like the physical appearance of your house, the physical appearance of your body affects not only the way you feel, but also your state of mind.

Bob: I'm not following.

Carol: Think of the houses you have lived in. Was there ever a time when one of them was a bit run down?

Bob: Oh sure. In fact, the first house I bought was what you might call a fixer-upper. It was a dump when I bought it, but it was all I could afford at the time.

Carol: What was wrong with the house?

Bob: Well, it had good bones, as they say. It mostly just needed to be cleaned up.

Carol: So there was nothing physically wrong with the house?

Bob: No, not at all. I wouldn't have purchased it if there had been.

Carol: And after you moved into the house? What was that like?

Bob: The first few weeks were awful. I mean, I can laugh about it now, but believe me, it wasn't enjoyable.

Carol: Why not?

Bob: Well, the house just looked horrible, both inside and out. The whole thing needed to be scraped and painted, and the land-scaping was overgrown too. It just looked like hell!

Carol: And what was that like?

Bob: It was a nightmare; much harder than I anticipated. At first I thought it would be easy: a coat of paint, pull some weeds, mow the lawn, put in some plants … no big deal. And in fact, that's what I did. In the end, it actually wasn't that big of a deal, and took about as much time and effort as I thought it would.

Carol: But?

Bob: But until it was fixed, I really hated living in that house. I would wake up in the morning and see the paint peeling off the ceilings and walls. I would leave the house in the morning and see the overgrown landscaping. I would look at the exterior of the house and see the paint peeling off the siding and the wood trim … Yeah, it really put me in a bad mood.

Carol: Tell me a little more about that.

Bob: Each day started off on the wrong foot. I became depressed thinking about what a dump I was living in. I was embarrassed at the outward appearance of my house, and I had anxiety from thinking about all the work I had to do to fix it up. I also dreaded going home each night and seeing that house. It really stressed me out.

Carol: So you fixed the house up?

Bob: As soon as I could. It took a couple months, but I got everything done. I cleaned the house, painted it, both inside and out, mowed the lawn, weeded the property, and planted some bushes and flowers.

Carol: Tell me what happened then.

Bob: Suddenly, I was in a better mood; everything seemed rosier and sunnier. I had a better attitude throughout the day, and was in a better frame of mind. I felt less stressed because all the work was done, and I finally lived in a clean, nice-looking home. I also noticed that people reacted to me differently; they were more talkative with me, and more social for some reason. Suddenly, everything just clicked.

Carol: Well that *is* interesting. Sounds like you experienced improvements in other areas of your life just by improving the physical appearance of your house.

Bob: Yes, I guess I did, but I'm not sure why.

Carol: Remember, Mind, Body, and Spirit are interrelated – each one impacts the other. A change in one area will impact the other two automatically.

Bob: But how did sprucing up my house make people friendlier towards me? I don't follow.

Carol: When you changed the physical appearance of your house, it impacted your mood in a positive way. Because your mood was better, you had a more attractive personality. Remember, people tend to mirror the emotions you display towards them. When you feel miserable, you project misery, and you attract misery back to you. In this case, you felt happy because of your house's improved appearance, you projected that happiness out to the world, and you attracted it right back to you. That is why people reacted differently to you, and were more sociable with you.

Bob: I'm beginning to see how this works.

Carol: The same principle holds true for your physical appearance. We tend to forget that many people respond to us by how we look, even if they do not mean to. This can actually affect how we think and feel about ourselves.

Bob: What do you mean?

Carol: Let me give you an example. Several years ago, I began to get a sense that people were not responding to me in a positive way – that they were ignoring me, or even shunning me. I looked through my clothing and realized I had not added to my wardrobe in years. Many of my clothes had become dated and even started to look a bit worn. As a result, I decided to update my wardrobe. I went out and bought some new clothes, which had the effect of modernizing my look and improving my appearance.

Suddenly, I felt better about myself, which put me in a better frame of mind, and actually lifted my spirits. I also noticed that people responded to me more positively and sociably.

Bob: But doesn't updating your wardrobe take money?

Carol: It costs less than you think. If you do not have a lot to spend on clothes, then go to a thrift store. Most will have your clothing size, and many actually have up-to-date things. Also, most everything these stores sell is in like-new condition. In fact, that is how I updated my personal wardrobe, since I did not have a lot of money at the time.

Bob: I see, but is it just wardrobe? Are there other ways I can improve my physical appearance?

Carol: Yes, you can improve your physical appearance in many other ways. Color your hair if you so choose. Get a haircut, or even a new hairstyle. To improve your skin, things such as taking vitamins, eating a balanced diet, applying moisturizer each day, eating avocados, and drinking six to eight glasses of water on a daily basis can make a big difference. Getting adequate sleep helps improve your overall appearance too.

It also helps to get a little exercise. Something as simple as going outdoors and taking a walk gets oxygen into your lungs and into your bloodstream, which makes you feel better, puts you in a better mood, and actually improves your physical appearance.

Bob: But some of these things are internal; things going on inside the body. They have nothing to do with how I look on the outside, do they?

Carol: We need to take care of ourselves internally, as this influences our outward appearance. For example, drinking water and eating avocados flushes toxins from the body, and hydrates and moisturizes the skin from the inside. Skin moisturizers also work to hydrate and moisturize the skin internally, which affect its outward appearance.

Bob: I'm not sure I follow you.

Carol: Let's go back to the example of your first house. Did that house have hardwood floors?

Bob: As a matter of fact, it did. I loved those floors.

Carol: And how did you take care of them?

Bob: Well, every week I would clean them with a wood conditioner. That kept them looking great.

Carol: What would have happened if you had not cleaned them with that wood conditioner?

Bob: These were older hardwood floors, so they would have dried out.

Carol: Exactly. Those hardwood conditioners work by actually soaking into the wood and moisturizing it internally, which not only preserves the wood, but also affects its outward appearance. Applying moisturizer to your skin works in exactly the same way.

Bob: Good analogy. Makes sense. So keeping up your physical appearance actually makes you feel better about yourself, which puts you in a better frame of mind. It also gives you a more attractive personality, so people will react to you in a more positive way. Is that correct?

Carol: Once again, excellent summary.

Bob: These Mind techniques aren't as obvious as the Spirit ones. What's next?

Carol: **Live your life regardless of your age.**

Bob: Here's another one that's not so obvious!

Carol: This simply means be happy to be alive, regardless of your age. Accept your chronological age, but do not dwell on it. It is what it is, and besides, it is somewhat irrelevant.

Bob: What do you mean by that?

Carol: Did you ever hear the phrase, "You're only as old as you feel"?

Bob: Of course.

Carol: What this phrase really means is, you're only as old as you think you are. Your state of mind regarding your age is the key to understanding what this means. I have spoken to many people over the years that still think and feel the same way they did when they were in their late teens or early twenties. There may be certain physical limitations as the body ages, but there are no mental ones. The mind cannot tell that the body is getting older. In fact, the only time the mind knows that the body is aging is when we tell it.

Bob: So what does that mean? All we have to do is think young thoughts, or tell ourselves we're young, and it's as easy as that?

Carol: In a way, yes. Remember, we are talking about Mind now, and age, just like many things, is a state of mind.[20]

Bob: I don't buy it.

Carol: Have you ever heard of anyone who has lived for an extremely long time? There are examples all around us. News programs regularly announce the birthdays of people who are over 100, 105, or sometimes over 110. Do you ever wonder how these individuals have managed to live so long?

Bob: Well, yes.

Carol: When I was working as a geriatric nurse, I encountered similar people, and I found that their long lives were due to a combination of things – some hereditary, some not. One of the things I found, though, was that most people who lived a long life *thought young* and were happy for each day that they were alive.[21]

Bob: So I just go along pretending I'm 18 years old forever? Do the things I did when I was that age? Climb trees and jump over fences?

Carol: Well, not exactly. As with all things in life, there is a balance here. Enjoy what you are still able to do, but be realistic about what physical activities you are capable of. Be sensible, and do not try to do anything foolish. For example, at the age of 84, my mother gave herself a hernia and put herself in the hospital by trying to lift a 50-pound bag of lime. She never accepted that she was old, which was great; however, she never balanced that thought with the realities of what she was, and was not, still able to do physically, and it got her into trouble.

Bob: Was she alright? Your mom, I mean.

Carol: Thankfully, yes. She also learned her lesson and never tried that again. So you should always think young, as that positively affects your Mind, Body, and Spirit. Just make sure you know what you physically can and cannot still do.

Bob: Okay, but how do I know when I'm overdoing the physical part?

Carol: Your body will tell you. All you have to do is listen to it. If you begin a physical activity, like starting to lift a 50-pound bag of lime, and it feels like it is too much for you, then it probably is.

Bob: So it looks like my tree climbing and fence jumping days are over. I don't feel like ending up in the hospital just so I can play teenager for a minute or two. But I understand, and I'll be smart about what physical activities I take on. Okay, what's next?

Carol: **Live in the present.**

Bob: What's this one all about?

Carol: It means you are not living in the past. Disengaged from the present; spending most of your time trying to recapture how things used to be. Nothing happens in the past. It all happens now, at this moment in time.

Bob: Longing for a simpler time, what's wrong with that?

Carol: It is fine to reminisce about how things used to be, and to tell old stories once in a while. But not all the time, and especially not when younger friends and acquaintances are around.

Bob: Why not?

Carol: For one thing, it repels people. Individuals who were not alive back in the old days, so to speak, have no reference point to the past, so they cannot relate to either you or your stories.

Bob: I guess I can see that, but how does that actually repel people?

Carol: When you talk about the past, you will invariably talk about how you have nothing in common with today's young people. And because you are only reminiscing about the past, you are not creating any common experiences with these young people, so this becomes a self-fulfilling prophecy. You eventually wind up driving them away.

Bob: Okay, but how does that affect my mind, since we have nothing in common anyway?

Carol: It is not just young people you wind up driving away. When you continuously long for what you see as a better time, you disengage from the present. It is almost as if you leave the current world, and mentally travel back in time. Since you are the only person who can live in your past, you end up living in a community with a population of only one person, and that person is you. You eventually become isolated from society, which can lead to loneliness and depression.

Also, when you live in the past, you do not appreciate all of the wonderful things that are present around you, which further isolates you from society. This can lead to more loneliness, and ultimately to further depression. It is a downward spiral.

Bob: But I like remembering the simpler times. You have to admit that communication was more personal, and the world was a less dangerous place, several decades ago.

Carol: It is true that the way people communicate has changed drastically, and the Internet has certainly made it easier for scammers and predators to operate. However, most of us look at the past with rose-colored glasses. We remember only the good times, and conveniently forget the periods when things were tough.

Bob: What do you mean by that?

Carol: Let's pick a few periods in history and I'll illustrate. Let's take the Roaring Twenties. Great time to be alive, right? So much growth and prosperity.

Bob: I don't know, but from what I hear, it was.

Carol: Well, that was just after the country emerged from World War I, Prohibition lasted the entire decade, and in 1929 the stock market crashed and sent the United States into the Great Depression.

Bob: Okay, how about the 1950s? A nice period in American history.

Carol: The fifties are indeed remembered as a time of optimism in America. However, the decade began with the Korean War, and ended with tensions beginning to build in Vietnam. Also, people began to fear that the nuclear arms race, and escalating tensions with Russia, would lead to World War III, which would end life on Earth as we know it.

Bob: The 1960s? The peace movement?

Carol: In 1965 we entered into the Vietnam War, and we had three major political assassinations: President John F. Kennedy, his brother Robert F. Kennedy, and Dr. Martin Luther King, Jr.

Bob: Okay, okay, I get it! So the "good 'ol days" weren't as good as I made them out to be. But today, we live with the threat of terrorism, and personal identity theft. So things aren't so great right now, are they? How can living in the present possibly lead to a healthier mental state?

Carol: Living in the present is about living in the here and now, being mentally present rather than being disengaged and living in the past. Being a part of life today, happening at this very moment.

Bob: I don't understand.

Carol: If you were to sit here thinking about your to-do list instead of engaging in our discussion, you would not be living in the present. Your mind would be off somewhere else, and you would essentially miss what is going on right now.

Bob: Oh, I see.

Carol: And the same thing happens when you reminisce about the past, you disengage from the present world to travel back in time, essentially missing everything that is going on around you.

Conversely, living in the present engages you with society and your surroundings, with what is going on right at this moment, which helps you avoid isolation and depression. It also helps you relate to, and learn to appreciate, the good things around you because you are actually experiencing them. Like going for a walk on a crisp autumn morning, or taking a drive through the countryside. That is how living in the present leads to a healthier mental state.

Bob: I guess I get it, but the past was a part of my life. I like it there.

Carol: It is fine to reminisce fondly and share stories about the past; however, balance that with living in the present.

Bob: Fair enough. So what can I do to live in the present?

Carol: There are two ways to live in the present. The first way is to remain in the present. That is, do not become so engrossed in the past – with what has been. Instead, push yourself to participate in the world today; engaging in the events, and with the people, all around you.

The second way to live in the present is to learn to appreciate what is better about today; what is present today that has improved your life. This will help you realize that there are benefits to being alive today; things that you have today that you did not have in the "good 'ol days." Modern conveniences, medical advances, and so on.

We will discuss ways that you can participate in present day life, when we talk about our next technique – **Push yourself to participate**. For now, let's focus on what is better about today.

Bob: So what do you want me to do, write down things that I appreciate in the world today?

Carol: Well, you could do that, but that is too similar to the other exercises you have already done, so there would be quite a bit of overlap with your other lists. Let's make this list a bit more specific to you. I want you to write down how your life has been improved by either modern conveniences, technology, or medical advances.

Bob: Okay, I think I understand, but I'm not sure what to write, or how to write it. Could you give me an example?

Carol: Sure. First list each item, then briefly write about how it has improved your life. Let me give you an example from each category. For modern conveniences, you might list cordless telephones. You could write that this has improved your life by allowing you to walk around the house while talking on the phone. For technology, you might list home security systems, which deter burglaries and give you a feeling of safety and security. For medical advances, you might list the Polio vaccination, which has eradicated Polio from the face of the earth, so you no longer have to worry about getting stricken with this debilitating disease.

Bob: Okay, I'll try, but what if I can't come up with something in a particular category, medical advances for instance?

Carol: You do not need to come up with an item for each category, the point of this exercise is to think about how things in the world today make your life better.

Bob: I see.

Carol: So take a few minutes and write this list up. We will discuss how to use it after you have written it.

To the Reader:

Can you help Bob complete this list? Go to Appendix B and find the section titled **"Live in the present."** Write down how your life has been improved by either modern conveniences, technology, or medical advances. As Carol said, do not worry if you don't have an item for each category. Complete this table before reading on.

Bob: I'm done with this list. So how do I use it?

Carol: Take this list and put it up where you can see it. Again, maybe on your bathroom mirror or on the wall next to your dresser. Add a periodic review of it to your schedule of exercises. Then, every morning, or whenever you have this exercise scheduled for, review the list to remind yourself of the things in modern society that have improved your life.

Bob: I see, but what does that do for me?

Carol: It shifts your thinking and gets you focused on the positive things that modern advances allow you to do. Ways that modern advances make your life better, and allow you to do things you could not do in the past. In short, it helps you realize that this is a good time to be alive.

Bob: Okay, so one final question. What about the past? The past is part of my life. What should I do to make sure I remember the good things from my past? What can I bring forward from that time into my current life?

Carol: You should make an effort to remember those things from your past experiences that helped you. This will allow you to remember the good things from your past without dwelling on what you thought were better times.

Bob: Makes sense.

Carol: And remember, you take your past with you wherever you go. It is part of you, so you do not need to worry about forgetting it. What you bring from the past into today's environment, and into the future, is your system of beliefs and values. These are timeless, and will never go out of style.

Bob: That's a lot to chew on, so let me make sure I've got it straight in my head. I need to live in the present to stay mentally engaged with people and society. I can reminisce, but mostly for my own enjoyment. And too much conversation about the past will drive people away. I need to learn to appreciate what's going on around me, and stay engaged with people and events taking place at this moment in time. I can bring my past beliefs and values with me into my current environment, and even into the future, which is a good way for me to stay connected to my past without disengaging from the present. Do I have it correct?

Carol: I could not have said it better myself.

Bob: Okay, what's next?

Carol: **Push yourself to participate.**

Bob: So we just got done discussing living in the present, and you said that pushing yourself to participate was one of the two ways to do that. Correct?

Carol: Correct. That is why this is a follow-on to the last technique. Appreciating modern advances definitely helps you live in the present. Another way to do this, however, is to simply push yourself to participate in life by going out into the world and engaging with people.

Bob: But what if I'm tired, and I just want to stay home?

Carol: We have all felt that way at times, even me. It is easy to sit at home and watch TV or movies. Indeed, sometimes quiet time by yourself is needed. However, you need to balance alone time with social activity – time with other people. For instance, sometimes my friends want me to go out to dinner and a movie with them. At times, their invitation comes when I am a little tired, and just feel like staying home. Even so, I usually say yes to their invitation unless I have a prior commitment, or have a cold or flu.

Bob: Even if you're tired? How come?

Carol: Because if I do not, if I consistently refuse, they will eventually stop calling and inviting me out. That has happened to me in the past.

Bob: Really? I can't believe that. You?

Carol: Sad but true. I lost a very close friend that way. We still keep in touch, but we are not as close as we used to be. It happened about 16 years ago, when I was still working as an in-home caregiver. The job was tiring me out, and I was contemplating retirement.

It started innocently enough. For years, my friend used to call and invite me to have dinner with her, usually about once a week. It was nice to see her, and we always had a good evening out. However, as the years wore on, being a full-time caregiver started to take its toll on me. The days just wore me out. Eventually, it got so bad that all I felt like doing at the end of the day was going home, flopping in my chair, and watching TV.

Bob: That sounds like how I felt for a while. So what happened?

Carol: Well, I started making excuses. I started telling my friend that I was either too tired to go out to dinner, or that I was not feeling well and did not want to get her sick. I apologized each time, and she said she understood. It went on that way for a while. She persisted, but I kept refusing her efforts.

Bob: So how did things turn out?

Carol: She eventually got tired of asking me to dinner, knowing I would almost certainly refuse. In fact, she stopped calling me altogether for several months. When we finally did resume talking, it was not the same as it had been. We are still friendly, and talk on the phone about once a month or so, but we never go to dinner anymore, and we are not nearly as close as we once were.

Bob: That's kind of sad. So if I constantly reject people's efforts, they'll eventually stop calling me?

Carol: Yes, most likely.

Bob: Okay, what's next?

Carol: **Do it now.**

Bob: Sounds like this has something to do with procrastination, but what does that have to do with mental attitude?

Carol: Well, procrastination clutters the mind and slowly overwhelms it, which can lead to stress, anxiety, depression, and a negative mental attitude.

Bob: How so? I mean, how can putting one task off for a day or two lead to stress, anxiety, and depression?

Carol: It often starts off with just one task. We put that task off, thinking we will do it tomorrow or the next day. If this continues for too long, then our to-do list keeps building and building until it becomes overwhelming. Our minds start to become cluttered trying to keep track of all the things we need to do. Procrastination can even have adverse impacts on physical health.[22]

Bob: Okay, I think I understand. But what about just writing things down? Doesn't that relieve the mind from being overburdened?

Carol: Writing things down helps, of course, but this does not prevent your mind from being overburdened. Your subconscious mind knows that you still have tasks to do, even if you are not consciously aware of them.

Bob: What do you mean by that?

Carol: Have you ever been sitting alone, quietly watching TV or maybe reading a book, and an unfinished task of yours just seems to pop into your head out of nowhere?

Bob: Yes, it happened to me yesterday. I had an issue with setting up automated payments for one of my credit cards. I'd been meaning to get it resolved, but just kept putting it off. I'd written it down, so I wasn't really thinking about it much. In fact, I'd almost forgotten about it when all of a sudden, it popped into my head out of nowhere.

Carol: Exactly. Even though you wrote this task down, you did not actually forget it. Your subconscious was still thinking about it and expending effort trying to keep track of it. You never really forget about an unfinished task; your mind stores it in memory until it is done.

Bob: So even if I write them down, these unfinished tasks lead to a cluttered mind? I can understand that.

Carol: And if this continues for too long, your subconscious to-do list becomes so big that your mind actually freezes. You have so many things to do, that you feel overwhelmed and do not know where to begin. It can be quite depressing and mentally draining.

Bob: I'm pretty sure I know what you mean, but do you have an example? Just so I'm clear.

Carol: Sure. Several years back, I was preparing to throw a large and elaborate holiday party. I had so many things to do: the house needed to be cleaned from top to bottom; I needed to polish the good silverware and clean the fine china; I had to plan the menu, do the shopping, then do the cooking, among dozens of other tasks, including decorating for the holiday.

Now, I could have started several of these tasks weeks in advance of the party, but I did not. Instead, I kept putting them off until it was almost too late. By then, my to-do list seemed overwhelming to me.

Bob: What did you do?

Carol: I froze. I did not do anything, hoping my task list would simply go away, but as you can imagine, it did not. I soon ran out of time, and had to cancel my holiday party. I called everybody and made up an excuse that I had come down with a terrible flu at the last minute and had to cancel because I did not want to get everybody sick for the holidays. I was so depressed and disappointed. It ruined that holiday season for me, and I had no one to blame but myself.

Bob: Couldn't you just have not done all of those unfinished tasks? Wouldn't that have cleared your mind?

Carol: I could have decided not to do some of the minor ones, but I actually had to complete most of the tasks or there would not have been a party. For instance, I had to plan the menu, or there would not have been a dinner. I had to shop for food, or there would not have been anything to cook.

Bob: I see.

Carol: As with my holiday party, you can leave some minor tasks undone, but you will need to complete most tasks on your list; they do not simply go away just because you don't do them. They are always there, weighing on your mind until you complete them.

Bob: So does that mean I can never leave anything undone?

Carol: Not at all. It is nearly impossible for most of us to personally accomplish everything on our to-do lists. In fact, as you periodically review your list, you may find that some of the tasks on it are minor, and no longer need to be done.

Bob: So what can I do about all those tasks; the ones I'll never get around to, or that no longer need to be done?

Carol: Well, if these tasks *are* minor, and you deem them unnecessary, then you can *decide* not to do them. However, you must actually make a decision not to do certain tasks, and either physically or mentally cross them off your list. You cannot just forget about these tasks; they will always reside in your subconscious mind until you deal with them.

Bob: What about tasks that need to be done, but that I just don't want to do?

Carol: You will always have tasks like these. Some you simply must do yourself, like renewing your driver's license. It is best to get these tasks done as quickly as possible. Scheduling these on your calendar will serve as a reminder for you. Other times, you will be able to delegate them to someone else. For years, I used to repaint my house when needed. As I got older, however, it became too much, and I hired someone to do it for me.

Bob: So do you always have to hire people so you can delegate tasks?

Carol: Not always. Sometimes you can delegate to a volunteer, like a neighbor who offers to help you with something you can no longer do. For example, one winter not too long ago, my neighbor saw me outside shoveling snow. He knew I should not have been doing that, and immediately came outside and offered to help. From that day forward, he always cleared my walkway and shoveled my driveway whenever it snowed.

Bob: But that's not really delegating, that's someone volunteering to do something for you.

Carol: Whether it is hiring someone, asking for help, or having someone volunteer to do something for you, the main point is to get these tasks disposed of as quickly as possible. Don't let them sit on your to-do list forever, or until you get around to them. If you let these tasks build up for too long, they will start to become overwhelming, and could have serious impacts on your mental, emotional, and even physical health. As I have said throughout our sessions, Mind, Body, and Spirit are interrelated; an impact in one area affects the others.

Bob: Okay, I see how procrastination is bad, so what can I do about it?

Carol: You can use the same technique that you probably used in your professional life; you can start keeping a personal to-do list. Simply write down the tasks that you need to accomplish, and prioritize them. Also, write down how much time it will take to complete each task, and when it should be completed. Use a daily calendar to schedule your tasks if that helps. Whatever works for you.

Bob: Do you have a to-do list form I can use as a starting point?

Carol: Sure, I developed one for myself several years ago. Let me give it to you now.

To the Reader:

Go to Appendix B and find the section titled **"Do it now"** for a copy of the To-Do list template. Feel free to customize it according to what works best for you.

Bob: Okay, thanks. I'll take this list home with me and start using it on a daily basis. What's next?

Carol: **Keep your mind fit.**

Bob: What does that mean?

Carol: Just like the body, the mind needs exercise to keep in shape.

Bob: I'm not sure I understand.

Carol: Do you like to exercise?

Bob: I wouldn't say that I *like* it, but I do try to exercise regularly.

Carol: Have you ever gone through a period of time where you did not exercise?

Bob: Yeah, I sure have. In fact, I usually go through periods where I exercise religiously, and periods where I don't.

Carol: And what happens to you when you do not exercise on a regular basis?

Bob: Nothing at first. Then after a week or two, I start to feel tired and run-down. Flights of stairs are no longer as easy to climb. And whenever I lift heavy boxes, they seem heavier.

Carol: Exactly. When you do not exercise regularly, your body quickly gets out of shape. The same goes for your mind.

Bob: So I should exercise my mind regularly, is that it?

Carol: Regular mental exercise is an important aspect of keeping the mind fit, but it is not the only one. Let me ask you another question. Do you have a healthy diet?

Bob: As with exercise, I go through periods where I eat very healthy, and periods where I don't.

Carol: And what happens to you when you do not eat healthy on a regular basis?

Bob: Same as when I slack off on exercise; nothing at first. Then, after a couple of weeks, I start feeling really sluggish and tired. It's harder for me to get out of bed in the morning, and I don't seem to have as much energy during the day. I also start gaining weight and feeling bloated.

Carol: So, keeping in shape physically is more than just exercising on a regular basis. Diet also matters?

Bob: Yeah, I guess so. What's your point?

Carol: Just as with your body, the same holds true for your mind. You need to exercise it and feed it nutritiously on a regular basis.

Bob: Wait. Are we talking about my brain or my mind? Food can't affect my mind, can it?

Carol: Not directly. But proper nutrition does support brain health. When your brain is functioning optimally, it supports all the activities you need or want to do, not the least of which is thinking clearly. So your Mind has a direct connection to your brain, which is part of the Body, and both a healthy Body and a healthy Mind lead to a healthy Spirit.

Bob: Makes sense. So how do I exercise my mind?

Carol: Well, as far as good mind exercises go, anything that keeps your mind mentally active will help. You can read a book, either for entertainment or to learn something new. Read the newspaper to stay up on current events. Do crossword puzzles, word searches, or other brain teasers. Keep a journal and write in it each day. Take a course at your local community college to learn a language or learn about other cultures. Attend lectures. Go to a concert. Join a discussion group like the Book of the Month Club. Go on day trips. Tour a part of the world you have never seen before. The list goes on and on. Basically, do anything you can to keep mentally active. You could even write a book.

Bob: Write a book? That might be a bit of a stretch. But I might like reading about other cultures. What about watching the History Channel or something like that? Would that count?

Carol: Absolutely. Anything that provides you with new information will exercise not only your mind but also your brain.

Bob: Interesting.

Carol: Yes. Studies have shown that cognitive health improves when you keep actively using your brain.[23]

Bob: I never would've thought. But what about the other thing you mentioned? What about nourishing the mind? Or is it the brain?

Carol: Actually, it is both. You want to nourish your brain, since it is part of your body. But you also want to regulate the type of information and energy you feed your mind. For instance, are you feeding your mind positive or negative thoughts? Are you just sitting around complaining about how bad things are and feeling sorry for yourself, or are you out in the world associating with positive people, positive experiences, and things that bring you joy?

Bob: Okay, I think I understand, but what can I do to make sure I'm feeding my mind positive things instead of negative ones?

Carol: Many of the things we have already talked about will help: not inundating yourself with negative news; associating yourself with positive people; and avoiding people who complain all the time. You can also perform many of the Spirit exercises we spoke about in the last session.

Specific ones that will help are: **Be thankful for what you have; Look at the beauty of nature around you; and Do the things you enjoy doing.** These specific exercises will feed your mind with positive thoughts and emotions, and positive emotions are some of the most nutritious mind food out there.

Bob: Okay, so I need to keep my mind active and exercise it just like my body. Is that correct?

Carol: Once again, excellent summary.

Bob: Okay, what's next?

Carol: **Keep in touch with time.**

Bob: What does that ...

Carol: I am assuming you would like to know what this technique means.

Bob: Yeah, I started to ask that, but figured you'd get to it.

Carol: Well, we all lose track of time, even when we are young, but as we get older, it gets worse. After retirement, it becomes harder and harder to remember what day, month, or even year it is, because we no longer have the structure of a work week to hold us to day and time.

Bob: I've noticed that myself. But how does losing track of time prevent someone from being in a healthy mental state?

Carol: A person who has lost touch with time feels disoriented, as if they are floating or drifting through their day. They do not feel engaged with the world. This is a very dangerous and negative place to be.

Bob: Could you expand on that a bit?

Carol: Have you ever been lost? As in geographically lost; not knowing where you were?

Bob: Yeah, I got lost in New York City once. I was in Manhattan on business and decided to go catch a Yankees game. I took a taxi to the game, so I really didn't pay attention to my surroundings. When the game let out, there were no taxis to be had, so I decided to take the subway. The subway station at the ball park was crowded, so I decided to walk a few blocks and see if I could get lucky and hail a taxi.

Carol: What happened?

Bob: Well, it was dark by the time the game let out; well after 10:00 PM. It didn't take long for me to realize that leaving the stadium area was a bad idea. I couldn't find a cab, so I just kept walking, trying to find a subway station. Pretty soon, I had walked so far that the stadium lights had faded into the night, and I couldn't find my way back. I also had no idea where the subway station was. From the look of things, I knew I was in a bad part of town. I was lost, and I had no idea how I was going to get back to Manhattan.

Carol: And how did you feel?

Bob: I was scared as hell. I had no clue where I was. I was nervous, disoriented, and my stress level was through the roof. I actually thought I might die that night.

Carol: So how did you get back to Manhattan?

Bob: Fortunately, someone on his way home from work saw me, realized I was lost, and took pity on me. Turned out I was only three blocks away from a subway station when he found me. He was a nice guy. He actually walked me to the station to make sure I wouldn't get lost again. I was so thankful that I gave him 100 dollars for his trouble, and I've stayed in touch with him throughout the years.

Carol: Lucky you. Well, you have accurately described the way a person feels when they lose touch with time. Disoriented, fearful, and stressed. They may feel embarrassed or foolish that they are not able to do something as seemingly simple as remember what day it is. And because of that embarrassment, they may also be reluctant to tell anyone they are having trouble keeping track of time, so they may tend to become even more isolated and depressed.

Bob: I know that feeling. I felt like such a fool for leaving the stadium area and walking around at night when I had no clue where I was. What an idiot.

Carol: That is what people who have lost touch with time say to themselves, and all of these thoughts and feelings have a very negative impact on the mind.

Bob: I can see that, and now I understand why. So what can I do to stay in touch with time?

Carol: Let me ask you a question first. When you got lost after that Yankees game, what if you'd had a map of the area, complete with the location of subway stops?

Bob: Oh, that would've solved everything. I would've known right where I was, and how to get where I was going.

Carol: Well, that is the same technique you use to stay in touch with time.

Bob: Use a map?

Carol: Yes, only it is a map of the day, month, and year, and it is called a calendar. Like a map, a calendar shows you where you are and where you are going, and that keeps you connected with time.

Bob: Makes sense. Throughout my business career, I used a calendar each day to remind me of things like meetings and lunch appointments. In fact, I was forced to look at my calendar to remind myself what I was doing each day … sometimes each week … or even each month.

Carol: Exactly. We do this so often during our work lives that it becomes a habit. Before long, we may not even realize how much we rely on our calendars to keep us oriented to time. The problem is that, once we retire, many of us simply stop looking at our calendars because we no longer need to. Before long, it becomes very easy to lose track of time. With nothing to do, and with no daily commitments or routine anymore, days blend into weeks, which blend into months, and so on.

Bob: Well I'll tell you, I stopped using a calendar after I retired. I'm one of those who used a calendar just because they had to.

Carol: I understand. So here is your chance to re-engage with a calendar.

Bob: Well, I've been using a small desktop type calendar to keep track of the days I do certain exercises. You know, the ones you assigned me. Does that work, or can you recommend something better for retired people?

Carol: Any calendar that works for you will be sufficient. That said, I do have a few suggestions. First, select a calendar with plenty of writing space; one that allows you to record appointments in a clear and legible fashion. Try to select a calendar that shows you an entire month on one page. Many office supply stores sell desk blotters that double as monthly calendars. These calendars are large, they allow you to write daily appointments legibly, and they give you a month-at-a-time view.

One other tip for using a calendar. Each night before you go to bed, cross off that day on your calendar. Just put a line through it to signify the day has passed. That way, you will always know what the current day and date is.

Bob: Okay, good advice. Anything else I should consider?

Carol: Yes, you always want to keep a monthly pocket calendar handy to keep track of things like doctor's appointments or lunch dates with friends. Keeping a calendar with you also prevents you from having conflicts about where you are supposed to be on such and such date and time. Today's cell phones come with built-in calendars, and keeping one on you is a very handy way to always have a calendar with you.

Cell phones also tell you the correct date and time; most of them display this on the home screen. Also, if you have a cell phone at your side, you can call family, friends, and even make appointments. It is a very handy piece of modern technology; something that makes life easier.

Bob: Okay, I get it, and I get the tie-in with your earlier point about how modern technology can improve your life. What's next?

Carol: **Continue to learn.**

Bob: Haven't we been talking about learning and keeping mentally fit throughout this session?

Carol: Well, continuing to learn is certainly part of keeping mentally fit. In fact, it is one of the best techniques for doing so. But learning is so important that it warrants its own discussion. Albert Einstein once said, "Once you stop learning, you start dying." So that should give you an idea of how important learning is to sustaining a healthy life.

Bob: But isn't it more difficult to learn as we get older? You know the old saying, "You can't teach an old dog new tricks."

Carol: That saying is somewhat of a misnomer. Taken at face value, it would appear to mean we cannot learn new things as we get older. However, what this saying really means is that habits people have adopted over their lifetimes are harder to change. This is because most people become set in their ways as they get older. If we put this into a saying, it would be something like, "Old habits die hard."

Bob: But what about all the scientific studies out there that back up the claim that it's harder to learn as we get older?

Carol: It is true that scientists once thought people learned more easily during their formative years, and that once a person was over 30, it was difficult for them to learn anything new. However, there has been research over the last couple of decades that is starting to counter this thinking.[24] Scientists are starting to realize that people can, and do, learn new skills throughout their lives. In fact, learning new skills is part of people keeping themselves mentally fit and mentally young. Recent research also suggests that one's interest – or desire to learn – may become more central to learning new skills as we age.[25]

Bob: I can relate to that. When I was in my late forties, I learned how to program a computer. I also learned about several areas of computer science: how computers work; how to design electronic circuits; I even learned the complex math behind all of it. Most people I knew were surprised that I was able to learn these new skills at the age of 49, but I had a genuine interest in the topics, and actually found some of the subjects easier to learn than when I was in high school.

Carol: I also saw this concept work in my own life. When I was in my mid-seventies, I needed to learn how to use a computer as part of starting this practice. I did not really need to do much heavy computing; mostly sending and receiving email. I had spent my entire career without using a computer, yet I was able to learn to use one because I was personally motivated. Today, I use a computer as part of my daily work activities.

Bob: Okay, so I see that I can learn new skills throughout my life. That's encouraging. But so far, we've only been talking about things I might have a keen interest in. What about more general topics? What's the secret to learning about those?

Carol: The key is to be genuinely interested in the subject area. If you are not interested in it, then do not bother learning about it. Instead, find something you are genuinely interested in. It is not so much *what* you learn, what matters is *that* you learn. This is because when you learn something new, your brain has to decipher and categorize this new information, and it literally grows new neural connections, further improving both brain health and thinking capacity. So the key is to keep learning. That is the secret to keeping mentally fit.

Bob: That's fascinating. So reading the newspaper every day will help?

Carol: That would definitely be good mental exercise, and it will help the brain develop, provided you are learning new information by reading that newspaper. It is this new information that helps the brain develop new neural networks. For example, if you were to reread the same book over and over again, that would not really help the brain develop. However, if you read a book on "How to Build a Chicken Coop" or "How to Learn Spanish in 30 Days," that would be learning something new, provided you have never done those things before.

Bob: Okay. I get it. So where can I go to learn?

Carol: There are several places you can go. For starters, many colleges and universities have evening courses. These courses typically cost money, sometimes a lot of money, depending on the college or university you choose. Community colleges usually offer adult education at affordable rates. You can also take online courses via the Internet, many for free, or for just a small fee.

You can visit your local bookstore and pick up a book on almost anything you are interested in. Even if you do not find the specific book you are looking for, the store can usually order it for you. You can also search the Internet for almost any topic that interests you; chances are good you can find a wealth of articles and research that you can read for free.

Your local library is also a great place to learn. You can look through all the different non-fiction books and periodicals available, and the librarians are there to help you find whatever you are looking for. The library also carries a wide variety of newspapers, both national and international, so you can catch up on current events from around the world.

Bob: Okay, so if I understand everything you've just told me, I'm never too old to learn. In fact, recent studies are showing that you can indeed "teach an old dog new tricks."

Carol: Well said. One more thing you should know. Studies have also shown that staying physically fit and eating a healthy diet aids brain health and mental function.[26] So, a healthy diet and exercise routine can actually help you learn more effectively.

Bob: Well, that's good to know. One more question. My eyes are starting to deteriorate, and I can't see as well as I used to. Does that mean I'll be unable to learn as I get older because of my declining ability to read small print?

Carol: Not at all. Aside from eye glasses and contacts, there are several other alternatives available to counter deteriorating eyesight. When my eyesight began to get worse, I started reading large print books and listening to books on tape.

If you do your reading on an electronic platform, like Amazon Kindle, they actually have a large print setting, as do most computer programs and Internet sites. So you do not have to worry about losing your ability to read and learn, even if your eyesight diminishes as you get older.

Bob: Good to know. Okay, what's next?

Carol: That's all I wanted to cover today. In fact, that wraps up our discussion of Mind.

Bob: That was great. Lots of useful information, tips, and techniques. And we didn't add too many new exercises into the routine, either.

Carol: Yes, I knew you were a bit concerned about that. However, most of the exercises occur during the discussion of Spirit, which is why I cover that section first. I also like to give my patients something they can start using right away.

Bob: Smart thinking.

Carol: Comes from years of practice with hundreds of patients and clients.

Bob: Okay, what's up next time we meet?

Carol: Body, which is the last of the three keys to unlocking the doors to happiness, health, and fulfillment. After that session, you will have all the tools you need to achieve your goals.

Bob: Sounds exciting. I can't wait. Well, I'm going to head out now. Have a nice evening Carol, and thanks again for today's session.

Carol: You are very welcome Bob, have a good evening, too.

Bob leaves Carol's office in a very positive state of mind. He has now completed two-thirds of the journey, and he is actually starting to see results. This motivates him to incorporate what he has learned about Mind into his daily and weekly routines. Bob is also energized. In fact, he has not felt this energized for quite a while, if ever. Through the windshield, he notices the sunset in front of him and marvels at its beauty.

Carol is quite pleased with how the session went; Bob seemed almost exuberant as he left her office. Still, the session was a difficult one for her, and she feels tired, nearing the point of exhaustion, something very unusual for her. She quickly shrugs off her tiredness and chalks it up to battling a very resistant patient.

The next session coming up is the easiest, the one on Body. This is well-trodden ground, and Carol is certain Bob will accept her counsel without much questioning or resistance. Her last appointment of the day complete, she decides to leave the office a bit early to get some rest.

As Carol walks outside, she is awestruck by the beauty of the sun setting before her. Her fatigue quickly vanishes as she marvels at nature's beauty and thinks about how lucky she is to be alive.

CHAPTER 6

⌒⟶

Body

It is 2:45 PM on Tuesday. Bob sits in Carol's waiting room; he is a bit early. As he sits quietly, waiting for the top of the hour, Bob has time to think. It has been two and a half months since he began his therapy sessions, and about six weeks since he began using the first of Carol's techniques in his daily life.

At first, Bob doubted whether Carol's techniques would truly work for him. Fortunately for Bob, Carol was persistent and convinced him to stick to the plan. He did, and it is starting to pay off. After about four weeks of practicing Carol's techniques faithfully, Bob is noticing a change. His spirits are up, and he is thinking more clearly and more positively. His negative inner self-talk is almost gone. He's even noticed his body seems to be healthier.

Maybe Carol is right; maybe Spirit and Mind do impact Body, Bob thinks.

Since BODY is the subject of today's session, Bob is more eager than ever to hear what Carol has to say.

It is 3 PM, and Carol appears as if out of nowhere. Bob, lost in his own thoughts, doesn't even hear Carol come into the waiting room to get him. Carol finally gets Bob's attention, and he rises out of his chair. He eagerly walks into Carol's office and sits down, ready to begin.

---------- ◎ ----------

Carol: Hello Bob, how are you today?

Bob: Fine Carol, and you?

Carol: I am fine, thanks. Today we are discussing Body, the last bit of ground we cover in our journey. I can see you are eager to get started, so let's get right to our list of Body techniques. There are eight key activities that can help you maintain a healthy body, especially as you age. Let me summarize them first, then we can discuss each one in more detail.

1. Go to a podiatrist
2. See your doctor at least once a year
3. Get your blood work done once a year
4. Have a doctor look at sores that are not healing
5. Have your ears and your eyes checked
6. Maintain good dental health
7. Keep active physically
8. Do things in moderation

Bob: Sounds like the typical "Do this to maintain good health" list I've heard countless times before. I know these things are important, but I feel fine. I'll start doing them when I start to have problems.

Carol: Whether you take these healthcare precautions or not is ultimately up to you. As I have said all along, it is all about choice; the actions you take are completely in your control. However, your goal, and the reason you came to me, is to learn how to achieve happiness, health, and fulfillment, correct?

Bob: That's right.

Carol: And I explained to you that there are three keys needed to unlock the doors to happiness, health, and fulfillment, and that the keys are named Mind, Body, and Spirit.

Bob: Correct.

Carol: And that all three keys must be used on each door to successfully unlock it; that using only one, or even two, will not do because Mind, Body, and Spirit are interrelated.

Bob: Okay, I see where you're going.

Carol: You are right that Body is well-covered territory. Indeed, medical science has done a very good job of analyzing and taking care of the human body. So well, in fact, that we are living longer than ever before. However, exactly how the health of the Body impacts the health of both Mind and Spirit is less well understood, and is just beginning to be explored by a small group in the medical community.

Bob: And my guess is, you are one of those professionals.

Carol: I am, and I would like to share with you some of my not-so-obvious insights. Ones that are particularly relevant to people of advancing years. Also, this third key is required to complete our journey through Mind, Body, and Spirit, so it should not be ignored.

Bob: Okay, you've convinced me. Let's go through it.

Carol: Good. We will begin with the feet.

Bob: The feet?

Carol: Yes. It is vitally important to maintain good foot health, especially as we age. That is why the first Body technique on the list is – **Go to a podiatrist.**

Bob: I know you have some point to this one. But I'll tell you Carol, once again, it's not so obvious. Why is this important to me, and how does it affect my mental health and my emotional state?

Carol: First and foremost, we rely on our feet for mobility. Most of the time, our feet are the only parts of our body that actually have contact with the physical world. We rely on our feet so much, in fact, that most of us do not even realize how important our feet are to us.

Bob: Okay, so our feet take us places, and they contact the ground. So what?

Carol: Since your feet are the *only* parts of your body that contact the ground, they support all of your weight. This can create an enormous strain on your feet, especially if you stand on them for an extended period of time. Have you ever spent all day on your feet when you were not accustomed to it?

Bob: Yes, during my first job, in fact, when I was a dishwasher at a hotel restaurant.

Carol: Can you tell me about your first few days on that job?

Bob: Well, I was 16. And as I said, it was my first real job. I worked an eight-hour shift, most of which I spent standing in front of a large industrial dishwashing machine, feeding it dishes pretty much nonstop.

Carol: And how did you feel at the end of your shift?

Bob: Forget end of the shift, I barely made it mid-way through without having to sit down; my back was killing me!

Carol: And how long did your back hurt you?

Bob: For the first few weeks, then it went away. I guess I just got used to it after a while.

Carol: While that is partly true, it is more likely that you were initially standing on your feet improperly, and your body had to compensate, which is what caused your back pain to appear. Gradually, you learned how to properly stand on your feet for long periods of time, and that caused your back pain to go away.

Bob: Really?

Carol: Yes, the human body is a connected system. A problem in one area of the body affects other areas as well. Sometimes that connection is obvious; other times, it is not. Have you heard the old song, "the foot bone is connected to the ankle bone, is connected to the leg bone, is connected to the hip bone"?

Bob: Yes.

Carol: Well, the hip bone is connected to the back bone, or the spine.

Bob: What's your point?

Carol: The way you stand on your feet can lead to pain and problems in other areas of your body, such as problems with your ankles, knees, hips, and even your back.

Bob: Okay, but I'm a grown man now, and I know how to stand on my feet properly.

Carol: Are you sure? As we get older, everything in our bodies, including our feet, becomes more fragile. Bones become less dense and more brittle, and joints start to become less flexible. There are 26 bones and 33 joints in the human foot, so this can become a very problematic area as we age.

Bob: 26 bones, that many? I really never looked at the feet as having so many parts.

Carol: They do, and certain areas of the foot become worn out and tired from years of use. This can be exacerbated if there are specific issues with the foot – like a corn or a bunion – that force us to stand incorrectly, preventing our feet from bearing our body's weight evenly. If done over a long enough period of time, this can cause issues in other areas of the body, such as back pain.

Standing improperly can even cause the spine to become misaligned, leading us to develop poor posture. This can ultimately lead to instability and imbalance issues, which greatly increase the risk of a fall. As you may know, falling is one of the most serious things that can happen to us as we get older. In fact, it can be life-changing, and even life-threatening, if we fall when we are going down a flight of stairs or a steep hill.

Bob: Yes, I know someone this happened to. So, are there any other physical impacts of poor foot health?

Carol: Yes. This is less well known, but poor foot health can actually affect our internal organs.

Bob: How's that?

Carol: Like every other area of the body, the foot has thousands of nerves and touch receptors that relay messages to the brain. If the foot is in pain, that can affect the messages these receptors send to the brain, and result in the brain sending false messages to other areas of the body, including our internal organs, which could then cause them to malfunction.[27,28]

Bob: I had no idea our feet were so important. I mean, we go through life hardly thinking about them. Until they start to hurt, that is.

Carol: Yes. Your feet, and their health, are very important to you, so make sure you take good care of them. Toenail health is usually a good indicator of overall foot health. If you notice a problem with your toenails, such as discoloration, odor, or thickening toenails, then go see a podiatrist.

They will check your toenails to see if this is an indication of a more serious problem. They will also check your feet for any skin lesions, soak your feet, remove calluses, trim your toenails, and apply lubrication to moisturize your feet – dry feet can become very problematic as we get older.

Bob: I see. So if something's funny with my toenails, is that the only time I should go see a podiatrist?

Carol: No. You should go to a podiatrist if you suddenly experience foot pain, or if you have chronic foot pain. Ideally, you will want to see a podiatrist on a regular basis. This becomes more important as you age. Regular checkups with your podiatrist will help you maintain good foot health.

You will also want to see a podiatrist if you have persistent sores on your feet. Having any sore on the foot can be particularly dangerous for someone who is diabetic. If not treated, such a problem could result in requiring special treatment, even amputation. Someone may not even be aware they are diabetic, so it is particularly important to pay attention to sores on the feet, as this could be an indicator of a diabetic problem.

Bob: Okay, I can understand that. But you've been telling me Body is connected to both Mind and Spirit, right? So how does foot health affect my mental and emotional health?

Carol: First, poor foot health may actually be an early warning sign of failing brain health.

Bob: How?

Carol: Your feet are the furthest away from your heart in terms of physical distance, and your heart has to work hard to pump blood to them.

Bob: So what?

Carol: As we get older, we can suffer from poor circulation – poor blood flow to our extremities. Blood caries oxygen, which is vital to maintaining healthy organ function. Numb or cold feet are indicators that the heart is having trouble getting enough blood to the feet. And since the brain is also a good distance from the heart, poor blood flow to the feet also indicates that the heart may be having trouble pumping enough blood to the brain.

Bob: So that can result in poor mental health?

Carol: Yes, it can. The brain is one of the largest internal organs in the body, and the one that needs the most oxygen to function properly. Poor blood flow to the brain deprives it of vital oxygen, which can decrease brain activity and lead to things like memory loss, slow thinking, depression, and even Alzheimer's disease.

Bob: Really?! Okay, you got my attention. So what can I do to increase blood flow to my feet and my brain?

Carol: Anything that increases circulation. Physical exercise is the fastest way to increase blood flow to the internal organs. However, go see a doctor if you are experiencing numbness or coldness in your feet, as this could be indicative of a more serious medical condition. After she rules out more serious issues, the two of you can discuss the best way for you to improve your circulation.

Bob: Makes sense. So what about emotional health?

Carol: The specific impacts of foot health on emotional well-being are less well understood among medical professionals. However, remember that the body is a system; everything is interconnected. Just as emotional health can affect mental and physical health, the opposite is also true.

Bob: What do you mean?

Carol: If you have an ailment in your feet – a bunion or something else causing you pain and discomfort – those messages of pain are relayed to your brain via your central nervous system. Pain causes you to feel bad. Chronic pain can lead to stress and anxiety, which can lead to negative feelings and a negative emotional state that lowers your overall spirit. See, everything is connected.

Bob: So foot health is important, not only for overall physical health, but also for mental and emotional health, and because of all that, I should go to a podiatrist on a regular basis as I age. Right?

Carol: I could not have said it better myself.

Bob: Okay, what's next?

Carol: **See your doctor at least once a year.**

Bob: Each year? Even if I feel healthy? Can't I just go when I'm not feeling well?

Carol: You could, but you risk missing a serious health problem. That is, until it's almost too late.

Bob: What do you mean?

Carol: In some cases, your body does not exhibit pain or other symptoms. This is commonly the case with liver disease.

Bob: Oh, I see.

Carol: So it is a good practice to see your family doctor at least once a year. This gives them the opportunity to routinely monitor your health, check your vitals, and verify that your blood pressure, weight, and heart rate are all within an acceptable range, and have not varied since your last physical exam. Your doctor can also check your cognitive function and assess both your mental and emotional states.

Bob: Mental and emotional assessments? From my family doctor?

Carol: Yes, your family doctor can do a routine annual mental health check, typically by administering a standardized question and answer test designed to detect early signs of declining mental health. For more in-depth mental assessments, you will want to see a specialist and have more extensive testing done, like blood work, psychiatric evaluations, and maybe even a brain scan.

Bob: Okay, so what do these mental health checks do for me?

Carol: Generally, a mental health check provides an assessment of your mental and emotional well-being. Specifically, mental health checks look for signs of depression, evaluate your thinking and reasoning skills, examine memory, and try to assess how you cope with daily living activities such as eating, cooking, and getting dressed. These tests are designed to diagnose mental and emotional health disorders such as anxiety, depression, schizophrenia, and eating disorders, among other things.

Bob: Sounds comprehensive.

Carol: They are. These tests are designed to differentiate between mental, emotional, and physical health issues, so your doctors can accurately treat the real problem.

Bob: So now I get the importance of the mental health check, but I still don't see how mental and physical problems lead to emotional ones.

Carol: As a person ages, they often experience many stressors, such as decline in functional ability, loss of mobility, chronic pain, and bereavement as friends and family start to die. All of these can result in loneliness, isolation, and distress, which can lead to severe mental and emotional issues, such as depression – a very serious problem for older adults. In fact, depression can also influence physical health.

Bob: Depression can actually influence physical health?

Carol: As I said, everything is interrelated. Mental health impacts physical health, and vice versa. Depression may actually make a disease worse, leading to greater depression, which leads to poorer physical health, and so on … it is a vicious cycle. Researchers have also found evidence of this bi-directional impact in patients with chronic diseases.[29] But this area still needs further scientific exploration so we can understand how specific improvement in mental attitude might influence a person's ability to heal from physical disease more quickly.

Bob: Okay, I guess I see why it's worth my time to go to the doctor once a year. So do I just go to a general practitioner for my annual checkups, and they refer me to specialists as needed?

Carol: That is usually how it works. However, you may want to consider going to see a doctor that specializes in caring for older patients – these doctors are called geriatricians, and they have special training in caring for older adults. They are like a general practitioner for older patients.

Bob: When should I consider going to a geriatrician?

Carol: You should consider going to see a geriatrician if you are on multiple medications and you are experiencing memory problems. Geriatricians have special expertise in assessing cognitive impacts of multiple medications, as these medications may actually be the cause of the memory problems. Geriatricians are also skilled at looking for early signs of dementia and depression, so you should consider seeing a geriatrician if you are worried you might have either one of these issues.

Consider going to a geriatrician if you have decreased mobility, as they can suggest measures to prevent falls, which are the leading cause of death and injury among adults over the age of 65. You should also consider seeing a geriatrician if you are hospitalized; people who receive care from a geriatrician while in the hospital tend to do better after they are discharged.[30]

Bob: So now I see how this all fits together. An annual checkup does more than just assess my physical condition, it assesses my mental and emotional health as well, and even checks for things like depression. After all, Mind, Body, and Spirit *are* all connected!

Carol: I think you are finally beginning to get it!

Bob: So, is there anything I should do before my annual checkup?

Carol: You can check your vital signs.

Bob: Isn't that what the annual physical is for?

Carol: It is true that your doctor will check your vital signs during your annual physical. However, people often become nervous when they go to the doctor, and this typically increases their heart rate, pulse, and blood pressure, three vital signs that doctors check. If you take your blood pressure at home, and it is a bit high when your doctor takes the reading in his office, you can show him the pressure reading that you took while you were in a more relaxed setting.

Bob: That makes sense.

Carol: Also, if you have hypertension, you will probably want to monitor your blood pressure regularly. Get a blood pressure cuff, take your pressure every day at the same time, and be sure to record it. Share these readings with your doctor during your next visit.

Bob: So nervousness at the doctor's office and hypertension can cause my blood pressure to rise. What else can affect it?

Carol: Emotional stress, increased physical activity, physical illness, and medication can all affect blood pressure. Monitoring it regularly will give you a sense of your average blood pressure over time.

Bob: Okay, but what are the vital signs, and what are the normal readings?

Carol: The vital signs are: blood pressure, pulse, respiration, and temperature. The normal readings are: blood pressure: 120/80, pulse: 80, respiration: 20, temperature: 98.6.

Bob: Okay, I think I'll be well-prepared for my next visit to the doctor's office. What's next?

Carol: **Get your blood work done once a year.**

Bob: I'm familiar with this. Whenever I do go for a physical, the doctor does a series of blood tests. He usually comes back and tells me that my blood work checks out fine, but I don't really know anything about these tests, or why they're important.

Carol: Blood is the primary fluid that gives life to both our organs and our tissues. It provides oxygen to the body's organs, regulates water levels in the cells, and removes waste from those same cells. Problems in the blood may indicate serious health issues like diabetes, anemia, a thyroid condition, or an infection, among other things. Your doctor uses various blood tests to check for these potential problems.

Bob: The doctors told me all that. It's just that I don't know what the tests are for, or how they work.

Carol: There are literally dozens of blood tests that your doctor can order, and they can be used to check for a range of things. For example, your doctor can use certain blood tests to verify that your various internal organs are functioning normally. Blood tests can even help doctors determine the underlying causes of deteriorating mental health.

Bob: Okay, that starts to shed some light on it. But tell me, do I need *all* of these tests every year?

Carol: Not typically, but your doctor will routinely order a standardized complete blood count as part of your annual physical. Doctors use this test to monitor your overall health. Among other things, this blood test detects problems with the immune system, monitors oxygen levels in the blood, and monitors blood clotting levels; important things for your doctor to check, especially as you get older. From there, he can help you determine which additional tests you might need. It all depends on your particular health needs or specific complaints.

Bob: Can you tell me what other tests they do, just so I know what's going on?

Carol: Sure. Other than the complete blood count, doctors usually order a basic metabolic panel, sometimes called a basic electrolyte panel.

Bob: Wait, what's an electrolyte, and what does it do?

Carol: Electrolytes are minerals in the body that have an electrical charge. They are important for balancing the body's water and pH levels – the amount of acid in the blood. They move nutrients into, and waste out of, cells. They also regulate nerve, muscle, and brain function.

Bob: Okay, so what does this test check for?

Carol: A basic metabolic panel is used to detect side effects of medication, as medications can affect electrolyte levels. In addition, this test is used to check blood acidity levels, which can indicate problems with kidney or lung function. This test also monitors blood glucose (blood sugar) levels, and helps detect and diagnose diabetes, which is more common in older patients. Also, unstable blood glucose levels can contribute to a host of mental and emotional issues, such as depression.

Bob: So blood work can find problems with the mind too?

Carol: Yes. Up until just recently, the main focus of blood testing was to detect issues in the physical body, but medical researchers are starting to see connections between adverse blood work results and poor mental health.

Bob: Fascinating, I had no idea. What's the next test?

Carol: The next test is the comprehensive metabolic panel. As the name implies, it is a continuation of the basic metabolic panel. Among other things, this test checks for risks of diabetes, liver disease, and kidney disease – things to watch out for as you get older. Your doctor will order either the basic or the comprehensive metabolic panel, depending on his judgement of what may be going on with you.

He will usually also order a lipid cholesterol panel. This test detects high cholesterol, which can sometimes be treated with medications or dietary changes. This is a very important test because early detection can help doctors manage high cholesterol levels in the blood. Too much cholesterol, particularly LDL or *bad cholesterol*, causes plaque to build up in the arteries over time, leading to heart disease.

Bob: I didn't know that so much could be monitored by having blood work done. Are there any other tests I should be aware of, or ask my doctor to order?

Carol: We have covered the main blood tests that doctors usually order. However, there are a few extra tests that become more relevant as we age.

Bob: Such as?

Carol: The first test is related to thyroid function. The thyroid is a butterfly-shaped gland at the base of your neck that sits on either side of your windpipe. It is a very important gland because it influences many vital functions, including heart rate and blood pressure. Thyroid problems are common in older adults, especially in older women, and are most frequently associated with fatigue and cognitive difficulties. More specifically, low thyroid function can indicate chronic fatigue, brain fog, low mood, depression, forgetfulness, weakness, and sluggishness.

Bob: Damn! So the thyroid is related to physical, mental, *and* emotional health?

Carol: Yes it is. Good thyroid function is very important, especially in older adults. Active thyroid hormones are essential for a happy mood, so it is vital to have the thyroid checked on a regular basis.

Bob: Okay, what's the next test?

Carol: A test for vitamin B12 levels.

Bob: There's a blood test to check for vitamin deficiencies?

Carol: Yes, there are several. But the test to check for a vitamin B12 deficiency is very relevant to older adults, so that is why I want to talk a little bit about it.

Bob: Okay, tell me about the vitamin B12 deficiency.

Carol: This deficiency is quite common in older adults, and it can be related to things such as fatigue, memory problems, and even walking disabilities. Having sufficient levels of vitamin B12 in our bodies is necessary for good brain function. Low B12 levels indicate a greater risk for depression, and can signal cognitive decline.

Bob: Interesting, and I can see the tie-in with Mind and Spirit too. What's the next test?

Carol: The next test that is particularly important to older adults is called a glycated hemoglobin (A1C) test. This test is used as part of an evaluation for diabetes or pre-diabetes. It detects average blood glucose levels over the prior three months, so it is often used to check blood sugar trends, and is a good indicator of how well patients are controlling their blood sugar levels.

Bob: Should I be asking for all these tests, or is my doctor going to just do them?

Carol: Your doctor will know which blood tests you need based on your medical history. However, you should feel free to discuss this with your doctor to make sure you understand exactly what tests he is ordering and why.

Bob: Okay, thanks for being so thorough. This is really shedding some light on this for me.

Carol: No problem at all. There are just a few more tests to cover. I want to make sure you know the ones that are important to older adults. The next test is called the brain natriuretic peptide, or BNP test. Contrary to what the name implies, this test is used to detect heart failure, which is common in older adults. BNP levels go up when a person's heart cannot pump blood effectively. This indicates that they are in some state of heart failure.

Bob: So does heart failure mean that the heart doesn't work anymore?

Carol: Not necessarily. Heart failure occurs when the heart cannot pump blood normally or effectively. Heart failure ranges from mild, to severe, to fatal – in which case the heart completely stops working. This test is extremely important, particularly for older adults.

Bob: Okay, good to know. Let's keep going.

Carol: The next two tests check for sufficient levels of magnesium and zinc in the blood.

Bob: What do those minerals do?

Carol: Those minerals are responsible for many things, but what is most important to know is that low levels of magnesium and zinc can contribute to depression and low mood.

Bob: Really?

Carol: Yes, so it is vitally important to monitor both magnesium and zinc levels, especially if you feel depressed or stressed, as stress depletes magnesium levels in the body.

Bob: Okay, got it. What else?

Carol: One last test I want you to know about; one that tests for the presence of cortisol in the blood.

Bob: What is cortisol?

Carol: You can think of cortisol as a stress hormone. Having too much of it in your blood can cause depression, low mood, stress, and anxiety. In addition to the serious physical consequences, like a heart attack or stroke, stress can also affect both mental and emotional health. So it is important that you manage the cortisol levels in your body and in your blood.

Bob: How can I do that?

Carol: Doing the Spirit exercises we already discussed will help you reduce your cortisol levels. Getting enough sleep and eating a proper diet will help too. Taking up a hobby, using relaxation or meditation techniques, exercising, and having fun doing what you enjoy, are also great ways to manage your cortisol levels.

Bob: Okay, got it. Anything else?

Carol: Those are the most important blood tests that are related to Mind, Body, and Spirit.

Bob: Okay, so let me see if I've got it. Getting blood work done is important, and I should have it done at least yearly. My doctor can determine if I need blood work done more often than that, depending on my specific situation and health needs. Also, in addition to monitoring the physical workings of my body, blood tests can find chemical imbalances, which often result in both mental and emotional issues.

Carol: Well said.

Bob: Thanks for going through all that for me. Now, I can actually talk with my doctor about this stuff. What's the next technique?

Carol: **Have a doctor look at sores that are not healing.**

Bob: Okay, this seems obvious, so why are you telling me this? What's the hidden meaning?

Carol: Sores are really wounds. When we are young and we get a wound, blood vessels around the wound expand to allow white blood cells and nutrients to reach it, which helps the wound to heal. This slows down as we age, thus slowing down wound healing. Diabetes, which is more prevalent in older adults, also slows down wound healing because elevated blood sugar levels contract blood vessels and harden arteries. In addition, skin loses elasticity as we age. And due to this, wounds can heal up to four times slower than they do in a younger person.[31]

In some instances, however, a wound might not heal at all, which could indicate a more serious problem. So it is important that you see your doctor if you have a wound that is not healing.

Bob: So slowing down I can see, but not healing at all? What causes that?

Carol: There are several reasons that a wound might not heal. Some wounds may become infected, or may be caused by an allergic reaction; both of which prevent them from healing. Some could actually be skin cancer lesions. Dead skin around a wound could prevent wound closure; this is more common in older adults. Poor diet and deficient vitamin levels, especially vitamin E, could also be factors. Excessive and prolonged dryness or wetness of the skin prevents wound healing, as does continued bleeding. A weakened immune system also contributes to the problem.

Whatever the reason, do not try to remedy these wounds by yourself. As I already mentioned, wounds that do not heal can indicate a more serious problem, and need to be looked at by a doctor so they can decide on the proper treatment. Also, try to keep from scratching, or even touching, these wounds unless directed to do so by your doctor.

Bob: I had no idea this was such a big problem for older adults. I can see how this affects physical health, but what does a wound not healing have to do with mental or emotional health?

Carol: Have you ever had a serious wound?

Bob: Well, sort of. Several years ago, I had an allergic reaction to a medication I was taking. It caused a horrible skin rash to break out all over my body.

Carol: How did that make you feel?

Bob: Physically, I was in a lot of pain. The rash really irritated my skin and made it itchy and uncomfortable. It was all I could do to keep from scratching it.

Carol: And how did it make you feel emotionally?

Bob: Well, the rash was on my hands and face, so it was visible to others. I was so embarrassed, that I didn't want to see anyone. I even took sick leave because I didn't want anybody I worked with to see me like that. I didn't leave the house until the rash had almost cleared up. And when I eventually did leave the house, I actually put makeup on my face to cover up any remaining redness on my skin. I just didn't want anyone to see it.

Carol: You just accurately described the physical and emotional situation a person goes through when they have a wound that will not heal. Only, it gets worse as we age.

Bob: What do you mean?

Carol: Imagine that instead of a rash, you had several open lesions on your skin. Imagine that they were covering your entire body, and were very painful.

Bob: I'd rather not.

Carol: My point exactly. A person suffering this kind of ailment, in addition to the physical pain, suffers due to embarrassment. They do not want anyone to see them, so they isolate themselves, and this can lead to loneliness and depression.

Bob: Okay, *now* I get it.

Carol: More than that, wounds that will not heal often lead to stress, which, in addition to causing mental and emotional issues, can actually further slow healing.[32]

Bob: That doesn't sound too good. So if I get a wound, is there anything I can do to help it heal more quickly?

Carol: Exercise can help speed up recovery because it increases blood flow to the wound. In fact, this is one of the most effective ways to accelerate wound healing. A study at Ohio State found that working out regularly can speed up wound healing in older adults by 25 percent.[33]

Bob: So what you're saying is, if I have a wound that won't heal, I should see a doctor right away, for the good of both my body and my mind. Correct?

Carol: Correct.

Bob: Okay, what's next?

Carol: **Have your ears and your eyes checked.**

Bob: Again, I can see the links to physical health, but the ones to mental and emotional health aren't so apparent. But I'm sure I'll see them once you start to explain.

Carol: Hearing loss, cataracts, and macular degeneration are common among older adults. If left untreated, they can get worse, which can cause people to have issues with common everyday activities that they take for granted, such as reading, talking with others, or driving a car. This can cause their quality of life to suffer drastically, which could lead to mental and emotional issues like depression, withdrawal, frustration, and embarrassment.

Bob: Okay, I already see the mental and emotional tie-ins.

Carol: Yes, and there is more. Hearing loss occurs in one-third of people ages 65 to 74, and in half of people age 75 and older. And studies have shown that older adults with hearing loss are at greater risk for dementia.[34]

Bob: So how do I know if I'm suffering from hearing loss? What are the signs?

Carol: There are many indicators of hearing loss: trouble hearing over the phone; trouble following conversations when two or more people are talking; asking people to repeat what was said; needing to turn up the TV volume so loud that others complain;

problems hearing because of background noise; and thinking that others mumble when they talk.

Bob: So is hearing loss permanent, or can it be treated?

Carol: While hearing loss can be permanent, it is often temporary and treatable. Temporary hearing loss is often caused by things like wax buildup, or fluid in the ear. Loud noises can also cause temporary hearing loss. It may even be caused by a punctured ear drum, which can result from infection, sinus pressure, or even putting objects in the ear, such as a cotton swab.

Bob: Those issues could apply to anybody, regardless of age. But what about hearing loss in people my age or older? I mean, when does that start to occur? Is there a particular age it happens at?

Carol: There is no specific age this happens at. Age-related hearing loss usually comes on gradually, so we often do not notice when it is happening. If you find that you are suffering from any of the indicators of hearing loss I mentioned earlier, perhaps your hearing is beginning to diminish, and you should go to a doctor for an ear exam.

Bob: Okay, but are there any age-related conditions that affect hearing?

Carol: Certain ailments that are more common in older adults increase the risk of hearing loss. Diabetes, high blood pressure, viruses, bacteria, a heart condition, a stroke or other brain injury, all increase the risk of hearing loss. Hearing loss can even be the result of certain medications.

Bob: I see. Are there any emotional impacts of hearing loss?

Carol: There are several. People with hearing loss tend to avoid connection with others. This can lead to loneliness, depression, anger, low self-esteem, frustration, embarrassment, sadness, grief, and fatigue, among other things.

Bob: None of that sounds like fun. So you mentioned that hearing loss is sometimes treatable. What are the typical treatments?

Carol: Hearing aids are the most common treatment, but they can be quite expensive. If you ever need hearing aids, make sure you check with your insurance company because they might be covered under your specific plan.

Bob: I hope I never need hearing aids.

Carol: You are not alone. I know people who refuse to put their hearing aids in because, to them, it is an admission of old age. These folks are self-conscious about how hearing aids look. But today's advanced hearing aids fit right into the ear, and are not noticeable by other people. Also, life is far better when you know what people are saying.

Bob: So besides hearing aids, are there other treatments available?

Carol: There are several. Surgery, certain medications, even special training can help improve hearing in people suffering with hearing loss.

Bob: So how often should I get my hearing checked?

Carol: At least once a year, more often if you experience issues with your hearing. Make sure you tell your doctor about any hearing difficulties that you have. If you have ear pain, or discharge, report that to your doctor as well.

Bob: Okay, so that covers hearing, but what about vision?

Carol: Maintaining good vision is important to overall health. Older adults are at increased risk for age-related eye conditions like cataracts, macular degeneration, glaucoma, and diabetic eye disease.[35] Generally, vision loss can negatively impact overall health, well-being, and quality of life in much the same way as hearing loss.

Specifically, those with poor vision are more likely to experience falls, isolation, and decreased independence. Also, things like reading the mail, going shopping, cooking, driving safely, walking, paying bills, balancing bank statements, or even reading medication labels can be problematic for a person suffering from vision loss.

Vision loss also impacts socialization. It can affect a person's ability to play cards or board games, for example. It can affect a person's ability to use a telephone, or even a TV remote. It can interfere with a person's ability to pursue their favorite hobbies. It also makes self-care more difficult because it affects mobility and heightens the risk of falls or other injuries.

Bob: I don't have any of those problems right now, but I can relate because my eyesight isn't what it used to be, and I'm a little depressed about that actually.

Carol: You are not alone in feeling that way. Vision is so important to us that its loss is often frightening and overwhelming, and can even be downright devastating. This has a huge impact on emotional well-being.

Bob: So I can see it's important to keep my eyes healthy for as long as I can, but how do I do that?

Carol: Maintaining a healthy diet will help. Make sure your diet includes fruits and vegetables such as broccoli, kale, oranges, and tangerines. Also, fish and whole grain foods contain essential fatty acids that aid eyesight, so make sure your diet includes these foods as well. Lean red meats and beans are also good to have in your diet because they contain zinc, which is a mineral necessary for good eye health. Vitamins are also essential for good eyesight, especially vitamins C and E.

Bob: So diet is one thing I can do on my own to improve my eye health. Great! But what else can I do?

Carol: Lifestyle changes also help. Wearing sunglasses when you go out helps protect the eyes from harmful ultraviolet (UV) rays. Quitting smoking decreases the risk of cataracts. Taking reading breaks every half hour helps reduce eye strain. If you have hypertension, reducing your blood pressure can help, as high blood pressure can cause blood vessels in the eye to rupture. Even doing eye exercises – where you physically move your eyes around by looking left to right, up to down, or simply moving your eyes in a circular rotation – can help improve eyesight. Of course, it is important to visit your eye doctor regularly to have your vision checked.

Bob: So how often should I see an eye doctor? Once a year, along with the other doctors?

Carol: At least once a year, yes. But more often if you have specific problems or symptoms. For instance, if you have any eye discharge, chronic itching, or redness in the eyes, you should see an eye doctor immediately.

Bob: So can vision loss be reversed or treated?

Carol: There are many treatments for vision loss. For minor vision issues, eyeglasses or contact lenses are the most common treatments. However, for more serious eye problems like cataracts, macular degeneration, or glaucoma, other treatments – such as eye surgery – may be necessary.

Bob: So all vision loss can be reversed?

Carol: Although there have been advances in the treatment of vision loss, it is not always possible to reverse it, especially when the eye starts to physically deteriorate due to age. However, it is possible to take steps to slow the progress of vision loss. For example, I am on an eye drop regimen for glaucoma and macular degeneration. I have also had eye injections to slow the progression of my eye disease before it becomes so bad that I cannot see at all.

Bob: So the key takeaway here is vision and hearing are very important to all parts of my health, and I need to make sure I maintain them as I get older.

Carol: Well said.

Bob: Okay, what's next?

Carol: **Maintain good dental health.**

Bob: I understand it's important to have strong teeth so I don't need dental implants or false teeth. So I think we can move on.

Carol: Well, believe it or not, dental health is important for more than just strong, healthy teeth. Oral care impacts the health of the entire body, and poor oral hygiene can lead to serious health consequences.

Bob: Interesting. So other than rotting teeth, what else can happen because of poor oral hygiene?

Carol: First and foremost, poor oral care can lead to heart disease.

Bob: Heart disease? Really?

Carol: Yes. There is a connection between gum disease and heart disease. For instance, people with periodontal disease are twice as likely to have coronary artery or heart disease.

Bob: Shocking! How does gum disease go from the mouth to the heart?

Carol: When a person who has gum disease breathes in, they inhale bacteria from their mouth into their lungs. These bacteria can eventually make their way to the heart, which is what increases the risk of heart disease. These inhaled bacteria can also lead to Pneumonia; older adults are more susceptible to this problem.

Bob: Damn! I'm really beginning to see how all these things are connected. What are the other health consequences of poor oral hygiene?

Carol: Diabetes is also an issue for people with poor oral health; severe gum disease hinders the body's ability to use insulin effectively. In fact, gum disease is linked to multiple systemic problems in the body, such as chronic kidney disease, rheumatoid arthritis, and cognitive impairment, among other ailments.

Bob: I'd really like to avoid all those. So what causes gum disease anyway?

Carol: Gum disease is caused by several factors: plaque, food left in the teeth, tobacco use, unhealthy diets, anemia, and cancer. High blood sugar can also lead to gum disease.

Bob: So that's gum disease, but what about tooth decay? Other than poor brushing and flossing habits, any other causes of tooth decay?

Carol: One thing that I will mention is dry mouth. The absence of saliva in the mouth can lead to tooth decay. It may seem like a small thing, but it is quite common. In fact, most of us have experienced dry mouth from time to time, so be sure to tell your doctor if you are experiencing chronic dry mouth.

Bob: Sounds like dental health is more important than I thought. So what can I do to make sure I've got healthy teeth and gums?

Carol: You mentioned one of the things a moment ago. Flossing. Floss after meals if you can, or in the evening before you go to bed. Also, brush your teeth and use a mouthwash two or three times a day. Try not to eat too much sugar or candy. Eat a balanced diet that includes calcium-rich foods; things like milk, cheese, and dark green leafy vegetables. Taking a multivitamin daily also helps.

Bob: So if this is so easy to do, and it's so important, then how come older adults don't take care of their mouths?

Carol: There are several reasons, but let me give you the major ones. The first one is isolation. As some people age, they tend to isolate themselves, and begin to neglect their hygiene as a result. Others simply lack a routine. Once people retire, they no longer need to stick to a schedule, so their routines can change. This can also happen when a spouse dies, in which case both routine change and isolation can occur. Another major reason is depression.

Bob: Depression? That keeps coming up in lots of places.

Carol: Yes. Depression is a serious issue for older adults. Depression lowers our sense of self-worth, which makes it harder for us to practice self-care, such as brushing our teeth. Depression is not just about being sad, it can lead to death if left untreated. The last major issue is forgetfulness; older adults can simply forget to brush their teeth.

Bob: So, this isolation, routine change, and depression business, is all this inevitable, or is there something I can do about it?

Carol: There are a couple of things you can do. First, try to keep socially active. That forces you to keep up appearance and hygiene habits, such as brushing your teeth. Also, stick to a daily routine that incorporates good hygiene habits. And see a doctor if you start suffering from depression or dementia so they can refer you to specialists who can help you.

Bob: So how does poor oral hygiene lead to mental and emotional problems?

Carol: It sort of snowballs into them. Poor oral hygiene leads to loss of self-esteem, which can lead to low self-image. And because self-perception is especially important to older adults, having a low self-image can affect social interactions. Also, social anxiety due to affected speech from loss of teeth can lead to stress and depression. There is more research needed in this area, but there is clearly a link between poor oral hygiene and a person's mental and emotional well-being.

Bob: Okay, got it. What's the next technique?

Carol: **Keep active physically.**

Bob: So I know physical exercise helps maintain a healthy weight, but are there other benefits?

Carol: Other than helping you to maintain your weight, there are many benefits to physical exercise. A strong and resilient body helps maintain the ability to live independently, and it reduces the risk of falling and fracturing bones. From a medical perspective, physical exercise helps reduce the risks of developing coronary artery disease, high blood pressure, diabetes, and colon cancer.

Bob: Colon cancer?

Carol: Yes, in addition to a healthy diet, regular physical exercise helps to promote regularity, which promotes good colon health. And good colon health is vital to the prevention of colon cancer.

Bob: So is that it, or are there other benefits?

Carol: Physical exercise also helps to reduce blood pressure in people with hypertension or stress. It improves mood, and provides a feeling of general well-being. This is largely due to the release of endorphins into the bloodstream as a result of exercise. Physical exercise helps maintain healthy bones, muscles, and joints – helping to control the joint swelling associated with arthritis. And as you mentioned, physical exercise helps us to lose and maintain weight. Our metabolisms naturally slow as we age, which makes maintaining a healthy weight more challenging. Physical exercise increases the body's metabolic rate and helps build muscle mass, making it easier for us to burn calories.

Physical exercise also reduces the impact of illness and chronic disease. People who exercise tend to have improved immune systems and digestive functions, better blood pressure, and greater bone density. People who exercise also have a lower risk of heart disease, obesity, and osteoporosis. In addition, physical exercise enhances strength, flexibility, and posture. It also improves balance, which enhances mobility.

Bob: It can actually improve balance?

Carol: Yes, the right kinds of exercise can help with balance, stability, and coordination by strengthening the stabilizer muscles in our ankles, knees, and hips. And both balance and coordination help reduce the risk of falls.

Bob: How about the mental benefits to physical exercise?

Carol: There are many. For starters, physical exercise improves sleep, helping us to awake feeling more mentally alert, energetic, and refreshed. And the endorphins released during physical exercise help reduce feelings of sadness, depression, and anxiety, which greatly improves a person's mood. Physical exercise also helps with brain function. It boosts creativity, and helps a person with multi-tasking. It also helps prevent memory loss and cognitive decline, and may slow the progression of brain disorders, such as dementia and Alzheimer's disease. Many of these benefits come from the increased blood and oxygen circulation that happen as a result of physical exercise.

Bob: That's a long list. How about the emotional benefits of physical exercise?

Carol: Well, as I mentioned earlier, the brain releases endorphins during physical exercise, which reduces stress and anxiety, decreases anger, and enhances mood. People who exercise regularly also experience more confidence and emotional stability.

In addition, physical exercise provides a person with a positive body image, and gives them a general sense of self-worth.

Bob: All of this is quite impressive. So the benefits of doing physical exercise look fairly clear. There's just one thing.

Carol: What is that?

Bob: I hate exercising.

Carol: That is understandable; I do not like it, myself.

Bob: You don't?

Carol: Not at all. For me, exercising is boring. I do not like the routine of it. Now by "exercising," I mean actually going to the gym and spending time running on a treadmill, running around a track, or swimming laps in a pool. No matter how hard I try, I just cannot get myself to go on a regular basis.

Bob: So that means you don't get any physical exercise?

Carol: Not at all. In fact, I get quite a lot of it.

Bob: How do you do that without going to the gym?

Carol: I keep very active. You can get exercise in more ways than just by walking on a treadmill. In fact, you can generally get as much physical exercise as you require just by taking a 15-minute walk through your neighborhood each day.

Bob: Really?

Carol: Yes. But you can also get your daily allotment of physical exercise in a variety of other ways. For example, I get a lot of physical exercise by cleaning my house and working in my yard. I use my vacuum for developing upper body strength. Mopping floors, gentle stretching to dust high things, raking leaves, pulling weeds, and sweeping the walks outside ... all of these activities use my muscles and get a lot of good results, for both me and my house.

Bob: What about things like playing golf?

Carol: Golf is a great way to get exercise and have fun doing something you enjoy. Just make sure to walk the course and not to use a golf cart, which would defeat the purpose.

Bob: But is it actually healthy for me to do things like walk an entire golf course?

Carol: If you are healthy, then it is generally okay to walk an 18-hole golf course since you would not be walking at breakneck speed. However, if you ever get a heart condition, or start to have trouble breathing, then you and your doctor should decide if walking an entire golf course, or even playing golf, would be overexertion.

Bob: On the topic of overexertion, what about sex? I mean, is sex overexertion for someone my age?

Carol: Unless you have a serious medical condition, sex is a completely safe and healthy activity for someone your age. And, in addition to the emotional benefits of sex, it is a form of physical exercise, and can be quite healthy for you. However, sexual activity does carry certain risks that you should know about and protect yourself from.

Bob: Risks from sex, at my age? What risks? Older women are past childbearing years, so there's no pregnancy risk there.

Carol: I am talking about sexually transmitted diseases, or STDs for short.

Bob: STDs? Isn't that only a problem for younger people?

Carol: Actually, no. While it is true that cases of STDs are the highest in younger people, cases of STDs in older adults have dramatically increased over the last several years, specifically cases of chlamydia, gonorrhea, and syphilis.[36]

Bob: Really? That's shocking. Why the sudden increase?

Carol: Several reasons. People are living longer, and living healthier, more active, and more youthful lifestyles, and sexual activity is part of that more active lifestyle. Medications have come out in recent years that treat issues plaguing older males, such as erectile dysfunction, making sexual activity possible again. And more seniors are living in retirement communities, where socialization and participation in social activities is encouraged. Also, many seniors have recently lost a spouse and suffer from loneliness. The combination of all these factors encourages sexual activity.

Bob: So that explains the increase in sexual activity, but why the increase in STDs?

Carol: Well, the mere increase in sexual activity among older adults accounts for some of it. Weakened immune systems – common in older adults – also contribute to the problem. In addition, by the time sex education began to be taught in public schools, many of the older generation had already graduated high school, and were either married or in monogamous relationships, so most older adults never received this knowledge – specifically, education about STDs and preventative measures.

Bob: So does that mean I should refrain from all sexual activity?

Carol: Not necessarily. But if you plan to remain sexually active as you grow older, you should always use protection, specifically a condom, as they provide the only physical barrier between you and your sex partner. You should also have yourself screened for STDs on a regular basis. Many STDs are treatable, and as with all diseases, early detection and treatment is the key to preventing long term damage to your health. Many STDs have no symptoms at all, so regular screening is the best way to detect and treat them before they pose serious health risks to you.

Also, avoid higher risk sexual encounters like one-night-stands and sex with strangers. Know your partner, and talk to them about their sexual history and any high-risk encounters they may have had. Ask them if they use protection and have themselves screened for STDs on a regular basis. Also, find out their attitude towards sex. Do they approach sex solely as physical gratification, or do they regard it as more spiritual and sacred? Do not be afraid to have these discussions with your partner. These discussions should be open and honest, and should be done BEFORE any sexual activity takes place.

Bob: I would never have thought I needed to worry about these things at my age.

Carol: Not many older adults do. It is a little known, little discussed issue, but it is growing in size, especially as the world population ages. I am glad you brought up the topic of sexual activity. It gave me the chance to cover the danger areas with you. Of course if practiced safely, there are many benefits to sexual activity, not to mention that it is a great physical exercise.

Bob: Okay, got it! What's next?

Carol: **Do things in moderation.**

Bob: This one sounds like it's going to be a buzz-kill.

Carol: Well, not as much of one as you might think. In fact, it can actually lead you to have a happier, more upbeat outlook on life.

Bob: I'm all ears. So, what does moderation apply to?

Carol: Moderation can be applied to almost anything, including overeating, use of alcohol, exercise, watching TV, partying, even brushing your teeth – you do not want to scrub so hard that you wear away that tooth enamel.

Bob: I don't do much partying these days. But I do still like to drink wine.

Carol: Just do so in moderation, say one or two glasses a day, maximum. As we age, it takes longer for our bodies to metabolize alcohol. The longer it stays in our bodies, the more toxic it becomes, and the more damaging it is to our internal organs, like our liver, our heart, and our brain.

Bob: Well, I certainly don't want to do that type of damage to myself, but it's good to know that I can still drink wine. So is there anything I should completely cut out?

Carol: About the only thing I would say to completely cut out is smoking. Smoking is dangerous enough to younger people, but it can have increased detrimental effects in older adults.

Bob: Okay, I understand the eating, drinking, and smoking things, but is there anything else that I shouldn't overdo?

Carol: Do all things in moderation, including things that are good for you. We usually think that doing more of something is better, especially if it is something that is good for us, like exercise. But too much exercise can strain both the muscles and the joints. The same goes for too much dieting; it could deprive the body of necessary nutrition.

Another example is wine. There is a lot in the news these days about the health benefits associated with red wine. However, consuming too much of it can cause inebriation, reducing both our judgement, and our control over our behavior, not to mention the negative effects of excessive alcohol consumption that we just talked about.

Bob: I never thought of that. So overdoing even a good thing can be bad?

Carol: That is correct. Working too much, focusing on a hobby for hours on end, spending all day checking email, web-surfing, playing video games … Most things taken to the extreme are bad for us.

Bob: Yeah, we did talk about the excessive cable news problem. I wonder why so many of us have such a problem with doing things to excess?

Carol: As a culture, we tend to think that if something is good, then more of it is better. And for a while, we are right. That is, until more becomes worse. Most of the time, we do not even notice anything is wrong until it is too late; everything is extremely good until it becomes extremely bad.

Bob: I'm not sure I understand.

Carol: Let me give you an example. Do you like pizza?

Bob: I love the stuff!

Carol: Was there ever a time when you ate too much pizza?

Bob: Yes, every time I eat pizza. I don't really know why that is. Pizza just tastes so good that I keep eating it. I eat, and eat, and eat. I'm still hungry, at least I don't feel full, so I just keep eating until all of a sudden, I get too full.

Carol: And what happens to you when you get too full?

Bob: It's awful. I feel uncomfortably full, like my stomach's going to burst. It usually takes a few hours for my stomach to digest all that pizza, then I start to feel better.

Carol: So is over-fullness the only negative consequence for you?

Bob: Unfortunately not. Since I retired, I've binged on pizza many times. It's my go-to comfort food, and I've put on a lot of weight because of it.

Carol: But each time you binged on pizza, you knew what was going to happen to you if you ate too much. You could have chosen to stop.

Bob: I didn't feel like I was overdoing it. I mean, I still felt hungry, and I was still enjoying the pizza, so I just continued eating. That is, until I became too full. Then I finally stopped.

Carol: Your story is a good illustration of why we have trouble with moderation.

Bob: What are you talking about?

Carol: As a culture, we have a short-term focus and tend to want instant gratification. This short-term focus is also part of human nature, and it served our ancient ancestors well. Whenever they found food, they took it immediately, not knowing when they would find it again. But today, we have virtually unlimited amounts of food available to us 24 hours a day, so this natural tendency actually works against us, and we usually end up with unpleasant results. To combat this, we need to exercise moderation.

Bob: That makes sense, and I can also see how the bad effects of something can sneak up on you.

Carol: Yes. Small things build up over time to create the issue.

It is never just one thing, or a one-time event. Take smoking, for example. No one is going to get cancer or die from just one cigarette. It is the quantity of them, smoked over a long period of time, that causes the problem.

Bob: Okay, I get it. But you haven't talked about the benefits of mental and emotional moderation. Is there such a thing? I mean, can someone be too angry, or too happy, or think too much?

Carol: Those are good questions. First, let's talk about emotional moderation. This might be better described as emotional intelligence, or the ability to express or feel emotions without being controlled by them. People in control of their emotions avoid taking negative emotions to their extreme. Sadness, anger, jealousy, hatred, fear, remorse, contempt … these are all negative emotions that can control and eventually consume you, if taken to the extreme. You do not want to control your emotions to the point where you suppress them, but you do want to be aware of them so you do not become a slave to them.

Bob: Why is that so important?

Carol: People who are not in control of their emotions tend to drive people away; they repel instead of attract. Think of a boss who constantly loses their temper, or a person who is upset all the time. Have you ever experienced either of those emotional outbursts?

Bob: I've experienced both, actually. My boss always seemed

to lose his cool over nothing, and my co-worker always seemed to get upset, almost to the point of tears, every time the littlest thing didn't go exactly as he had planned. I felt so uncomfortable around both of them that I wanted nothing to do with either of them.

Carol: Well, as humans, we crave stability. It makes us feel centered, like we are on solid ground. When we are in the presence of someone who lets their emotions swing wildly out of control, we feel unsettled, which in turn can make us feel stressed or anxious.

Bob: I can definitely see that. Whenever my boss yelled at me, I felt stressed, and I just wanted to get away from him. The same went for my co-worker who got upset all the time. It made me anxious, and I just wanted to get away from him.

Carol: Exactly. These negative mental and emotional impacts that you felt are a direct result of other people's inability to control their emotions.

Bob: Okay, I get the picture. So I see the benefits of moderating negative emotions. What about joy and happiness? Should they be moderated too?

Carol: Joy and happiness are not emotions that we typically need to moderate. If you are happy and joyful, this will only add to your well-being. Just remember to be aware of the reason for your happiness. If you know why you are happy, then you will be able to maintain that happiness.

Bob: Okay, that covers the emotional benefits of moderation, but what about the mental benefits?

Carol: Earlier, you asked me if it was possible for someone to think too much. While it is generally not possible to think too much, it is possible to think too long.

Bob: What do you mean?

Carol: During your career, did you ever encounter a problem that seemed unsolvable, even after you spent hours on it?

Bob: Yeah, several times. But the one that comes to mind was from early in my career. I was working late one night, trying to reconcile a bank statement for an upcoming financial audit. That particular account had not been reconciled for several months, so it was a mess. I worked late into the evening trying to figure it out, but I just couldn't seem to get it. Finally, around midnight, I gave up and went home.

Carol: So did you continue to work on the problem the next morning?

Bob: Actually, I figured out what was wrong on the drive home. It just hit me all of a sudden. I finished the bank statement reconciliation as soon as I got home; took me only fifteen minutes.

Carol: And that is the benefit of mental moderation.

Bob: What do you mean?

Carol: As an organ, the brain is the largest consumer of energy in the human body, and the brain consumes more energy during the thinking process than at any other time. In fact, after only twenty minutes of sustained thinking, the brain becomes depleted of energy and needs to be recharged. That is why periods of prolonged intense thinking tend to wear people out.

Bob: So what does that have to do with mental moderation?

Carol: Moderating the period of time you spend thinking – taking a mental break every half hour or so – helps refresh your mental alertness. Very often, we fail to solve a problem even after thinking about it for hours, then find a solution when we step away from it for a short while. Just like how you figured out the problem with your bank statement reconciliation on your drive home.

Bob: I see.

Carol: And this principle works with more than just problem solving. Taking short breaks during an extended study session helps increase the amount of material that is retained in memory. So mental moderation is useful, not only for improved thinking, but also for improved memory.

Bob: That's interesting. I can certainly see the benefits of emotional and mental moderation, and the physical ones too. I just have one question on the physical aspects of moderation.

Carol: Okay.

Bob: How can I practice moderation without it becoming a downer or feeling like a chore; like I am depriving myself?

Carol: You can do that by seeing the *value* of moderation. Remember the positive benefits you will get as a result of moderation, and do not look at it as a chore. This goes back to the glass half full theory; you want to look at the positive side of it.

Bob: That makes sense. I used to do something similar when I was trying to lose weight. For years, I looked at weight loss as a chore; I always seemed to have more weight to lose, and it was depressing. Then, I tried something different. I started visualizing the benefits of a fit body, and the good health I would enjoy once I achieved my weight loss goals.

That changed everything, and allowed me to make better choices with my food and alcohol consumption. All of a sudden, I didn't feel like I was depriving myself. I just felt like I was making the same choices that my *healthier self* would make. And it worked, too; I reached my weight loss goal, and I felt happier and healthier for it.

Carol: Exactly. Practicing moderation is key to keeping you happy and healthy, especially as you age.

Bob: Okay, that was useful. What's next?

Carol: That is all I have for today. I will walk you out to the receptionist so we can set up your final appointment.

Bob: Wow, that went fast! I can't believe we're almost done.

Carol: Yes, this was our last working session. We have one more to go. Our final session will let me see how you are progressing, and will give you the opportunity to ask any final questions before our journey officially ends.

Bob: Sounds good, so next week then, same time?

Carol: Actually, our final appointment will be three weeks from today.

Bob: Three weeks, why so long?

Carol: Well, I usually schedule this appointment for two weeks after our final working session, but I have a doctor's appointment that day, and will be out of the office that afternoon.

Bob: I hope it's nothing serious.

Carol: Well, I have been feeling a bit fatigued over the past several weeks. At first, I thought it was just the job that was tiring me out, but this fatigue has persisted for well over a month now.

Bob: Oh, God! I hope I didn't wear you out, Carol.

Carol: Not at all, Bob. I think it's just because I'm getting up there in years. I'm just going to have some blood work and tests done so the doctors can figure out what's causing my fatigue. I will be back at work and ready to go the next time we meet.

Bob: I'll say a prayer for you, Carol, and I'll keep you in my thoughts and send you positive wishes.

Carol: Thanks Bob, I appreciate the thoughts.

Bob: Have a good evening Carol, and take care of yourself.

Carol: Thanks Bob, you have a good evening as well.

———⊚———

Bob is nervous as he drives home. *I hope it's nothing serious,* he thinks. *Still, Carol seemed confident that it was something minor, so there's probably nothing to worry about.* With that thought firmly planted in his mind, Bob's nervousness disappears by the time he reaches home.

———⊚———

The next three weeks pass quickly for Bob. The day before his next appointment, his phone rings. It's the receptionist from Carol's office, who explains she will need to cancel his upcoming appointment.

"Carol has become sick," the receptionist explains, "and has had to take a break from her practice."

The receptionist also says she's not sure how long Carol will be out, but tells Bob she will contact him to reschedule once Carol returns to her practice.

After he hangs up the phone, Bob gets a sinking feeling in the pit of his stomach. Something is not right!

CHAPTER 7

Crisis

Carol is thinking about Bob; wondering how he is doing. She has given him her home and cell phone numbers so he can contact her just in case he needs encouragement. She does not usually do this with her patients, but feels a need to do so for Bob, as she senses he is still fragile and in danger of backsliding. Carol absolutely hates to lose even one patient, so she makes this unusual gesture for Bob.

Bob lets a week go by. All he wants to do is call Carol to find out what's going on, but he tries to let her rest. After a week, Bob cannot resist any longer, and picks up the phone to call her. The phone rings once, rings a second time, then a third. Just when Bob gets ready to hang up, thinking that no one is home, someone picks up the phone. A faint, barely audible, and depressed-sounding voice speaks.

———⊛———

Carol: Hel ... Hello?

Bob: Carol?

Carol: Yes, this is Carol, who is this?

Bob: Carol, it's Bob.

Carol: Bob? Oh, Bob. My patient, from the office?

Bob: Yes, that's right.

Carol: I'm sorry. I didn't recognize your voice.

Bob: That's okay. I'm sorry to bother you.

Carol: Not at all Bob, that's why I gave you my home number. How are you doing? Do you need any help with your exercises, or do you have any questions for me?

Bob: Oh no, not at all. I was calling to see how you were doing. I got worried when your receptionist called to cancel our appointment the other week.

Carol: Yes, I'm sorry about that.

Bob: Not at all. She told me you were sick, so no apologies necessary. I was just calling to see how you were.

Carol: Unfortunately, I'm not doing so well.

Bob: What's wrong? What is it?

Carol: I'm afraid I have lung cancer.

Bob: Oh my God ... NO!

Carol: Yes, that's why I've been so fatigued these past few weeks.

Bob: How do they know it's lung cancer? I mean, are they sure?

Carol: I mentioned to the doctors that I had been unusually fatigued for the past month or so. They did a complete battery of tests on me – blood work, chest X-rays, the works. They spotted something they didn't like on my chest X-ray, so they took a lung biopsy, and it came back positive.

Bob: Carol, I'm so sorry.

Carol: Thank you. Fortunately, they caught it early. It's in stage 1, and it's treatable.

Bob: Forgive me for asking, but how did you get lung cancer? You're such a healthy and vibrant woman.

Carol: I got it from smoking.

Bob: You, a smoker? I never would've guessed.

Carol: Yes, unfortunately it's true. In fact, I've been a smoker for most of my life; a heavy smoker at some points.

Bob: When did you begin smoking?

Carol: When I was a teenager. All the negative effects of smoking, like the link to lung and heart disease, hadn't come out yet. Most of the kids in my high school thought smoking was chic and sophisticated, and all of the *in crowd* smoked … it was the thing to do.

Bob: And you continued from there to the present day?

Carol: Yes. Though my smoking habits changed over the years, I remained a lifelong smoker, right up to this very day, at least up to the day the doctors told me I have lung cancer. I haven't touched a cigarette since. Anyway, I continued smoking through high school into my twenties. It was the same as in high school, all the *in crowd* smoked; it was the thing to do at nightclubs and restaurants, and it made me feel so sophisticated. Then, when I started working as a nurse, I used smoking to steady my nerves; it relaxed me and decreased my stress levels. There was a time when I even considered smoking a *healthy* habit.

Bob: Healthy, really?

Carol: Yes, you may be a bit too young to remember, but tobacco companies used to run ads with doctors who would recommend certain cigarette brands. Anyway, I continued to increase my smoking habit until I eventually reached two packs a day, then all of the evidence linking smoking to lung and heart disease started to come out.

Bob: Did you try to quit?

Carol: Several times throughout the next three decades. I knew smoking was bad for me, and the evidence of severe health risks started to mount. By then, however, it was a well ingrained habit. I was still working as a nurse back then, and smoking did help steady my nerves and reduce my stress levels. So I kept on smoking throughout the rest of my nursing career.

Bob: Did you quit after you retired?

Carol: I tried again, but it was just too difficult. I also was continuing to work as an independent in-home caregiver. While I truly loved my work, it was stressful at times, and I used cigarettes as a way to relieve the stress.

Bob: And how about when you retired from that and started your current practice?

Carol: I continued to smoke, but I was able to reduce my habit to a half a pack a day. I also switched to slim cigarettes because I felt they were less harmful than regular cigarettes, but they may have actually been just as harmful. Still, by that time, the damage was done.

Bob: I'm sorry to hear that Carol, but you mentioned your cancer is treatable. That's good news, right? So, what are your treatment options?

Carol: There are three main treatments for my type of lung cancer: chemotherapy, radiation therapy, and surgery. All have their benefits, and all have their drawbacks.

Bob: Do you feel up to telling me a little bit about each treatment?

Carol: I think I can manage. The first option is chemotherapy. It's been around since World War I, and is the most common form of cancer treatment. In fact, it's the one that doctors recommend most of the time. The major downside is that chemotherapy drugs are basically poison; they cure the disease by killing the patient. Side effects range from nausea, vomiting, and hair loss, to organ damage, and even death.

Bob: Geez! Sorry, I don't mean to sound judgmental about any treatment option, but that sounds pretty awful.

Carol: It is. Effective, but extremely unpleasant.

Bob: What about radiation therapy?

Carol: Like chemotherapy, radiation therapy has been around for over 100 years. It works by damaging the DNA of the cancerous cells, causing their death. Unlike chemotherapy, radiation therapy is localized; the radiation is targeted only at the specific cancerous tumor.

Bob: That sounds a lot better than chemotherapy. Any downsides?

Carol: Well, radiation therapy does have some side effects; fatigue and skin irritation are the most common ones. However, radiation therapy could also lead to heart disease. In addition, it could cause issues such as dry mouth, dry eyes, and could even affect the taste buds. This could lead to a greatly reduced quality of life, which is a major consideration for me.

Bob: What about surgery?

Carol: Surgery is actually the oldest form of cancer treatment; it literally removes cancer from the body by physically removing the cancerous tumor.

Bob: That sounds like a winner to me.

Carol: Well, there are risks and side effects to consider. The main risk has to do with my age. Surgery for anyone my age is quite risky, and could even lead to death. There are also several side effects to surgery: pain, fatigue, appetite loss, bleeding, infection, and even organ dysfunction. What's more, the doctors are not sure if my cancer is even operable. They will have to do some more exploration before they can even tell me if surgery is an option.

Bob: I guess I spoke too soon. Are there any other options?

Carol: There are some other alternatives, but those are the main ones I am considering, and I need to decide on an option quickly.

Bob: What do you mean? Why?

Carol: Cancerous cells are created more rapidly than normal healthy cells, which is why cancer is such a dangerous disease. If left untreated, the cancerous cells eventually take over the organ they live in, and mutate it until it ceases to function. My doctors tell me the sooner I decide on a treatment option, the better.

Bob: I'm so sorry Carol. I wish there was a better option available for you.

Carol: Thanks. I do as well. I wish I had not started smoking all those years ago, and I certainly wish I had quit a long time ago. But what's done is done.

Bob: What are you going to do?

Carol: I don't know, Bob. I don't want to be infirm, and I don't want to live the rest of my life in a nursing home, or worse, in a hospital bed, alone, with only the nurses to keep me company. I just don't feel like there's a good option for me. I'm scared, and I don't know what to do.

Bob: I wish there was something I could say or do to make it better.

Carol: Your call helped. It was nice of you to check in on me ... I'm getting a bit tired now, the cancer and the stress of the diagnosis have really worn me out. If you'll excuse me, I think I'll go lay down for a little while and rest.

Bob: Okay, get some rest, and please take care of yourself; you'll be in my thoughts and prayers.

Carol: Thank you again for your call Bob, that was very nice of you. Call me if you need anything else.

Bob: Okay, thanks, but I'll try not to bother you if I don't need to.

Carol: Thanks Bob, have a good evening.

Bob: You too, Carol.

———— ⊚ ————

Bob hangs up the phone and sits motionless, as if in shock. He has never heard Carol proclaim her fear for anything. That's one of the things he loves about her. To Bob, Carol seemed invincible.

Here's a woman well into her eighties, he thinks, *who's going to work each day, helping people live better lives, and doing the work she genuinely loves. If a woman like that can be brought down by cancer, if her confidence can be shattered, if doom, fear, uncertainty, and doubt can overpower her, even though she is doing everything right, then what chance do I have?*

Suddenly, Bob feels his anxiety start to reemerge. He skips the rest of his daily exercises and heads to the bar.

CHAPTER 8

c⟳

Bob's Doom Reemerges

Bob sits quietly on his sofa, watching TV. He has a glass of wine in front of him, and an open bottle of wine on the kitchen counter that he is using to refill his glass whenever it gets too low. It has been a week since he spoke with Carol. The week has passed quickly, almost without Bob noticing. He has spent the majority of the week sitting in front of his television set with a perpetually full glass of wine.

Bob hasn't left his house much, except to go out to his favorite bar to get a drink and a bite to eat. But mostly, he stays in and orders pizza whenever he gets hungry. His kitchen is full of pizza boxes, some with half eaten pizza that has gotten too cold and unappetizing for Bob to finish. In fact, there are so many half-eaten pizzas in the kitchen that his house is beginning to smell like a pizza parlor, except not in a good way.

He has all but forgotten about his exercises. It has been almost a week since he has even looked at his calendar to see which ones he should be doing. It's almost as if Bob never went to therapy at all.

Just as Bob is about to get up to refill his wine glass, the phone rings. Slowly, he grabs the remote, puts the TV on mute, gets up from his chair, and shuffles across the room to answer it. It's Ted, Bob's closest friend, calling to check in on him.

Bob: Hello?

Ted: Hi Bob, this is Ted.

Bob: Oh, hi Ted.

Ted: Gosh, you sound a bit dejected, what happened? The last time we spoke you sounded absolutely giddy, almost like a little child.

Bob: Yes, that's when I was in therapy, but I'm not wasting my time with that anymore.

Ted: Why? You seemed to be making real progress with your therapist, Carol's her name, right? What happened? Why aren't you in therapy anymore?

Bob: I just found out my therapist, I mean Carol, has been diagnosed with lung cancer.

Ted: Oh my God! That's horrible! Is she okay? I mean, of course she's not okay if she has cancer. I mean, how serious is it? Do they know how she got it?

Bob: Yeah. Carol's been a lifelong smoker, a heavy smoker at times, so they think that's how she got it. She says they caught it early, and it's only stage 1, but cancer is cancer, you know; there's no cure for it. So yeah, I would say it's serious.

Ted: Well, what is she going to do?

Bob: The doctors gave her three treatment options; two and a half really. They don't know if the third one is viable yet. None of the options sound all that good to me. So, really, what choice does she have? She's probably going to die.

Ted: You don't know that for a fact, Bob.

Bob: Really? I spoke with Carol on the phone last week. She sounded frail and weak. She also sounded depressed and dejected; the brightness in her voice was gone. It was as if Doom came by and knocked the wind out of her sails, or worse, punched her hard in the gut when she wasn't looking. What's worse is that she told me she's scared. Can you believe it? A woman like that, my mentor, my hero ... scared.

That really shook me, Ted. If a woman who's that strong, that resilient, that full of life, can have it taken away, then what chance do I have? Maybe I was right all along, that our fate is pre-written in stone; that our destiny has been pre-determined for us, and there's nothing we can do but accept it. So what's the point of pretending like I have some choice in the matter? Look at what happened to Carol through no fault of her own.

Ted: Now Bob, I know this will seem a bit harsh, but Carol had a hand in this.

Bob: What do you mean by that? No she didn't! You think she voluntarily brought lung cancer on herself … on purpose? If you think that, then I think you're crazy!

Ted: Bob, you said it yourself. Carol has been a lifelong smoker, and she's also a medical professional. The dangers of smoking have been known, at least in the medical profession, since the mid-sixties. Carol undoubtedly knew about the dangers of smoking, and certainly knew that there was a link between cigarette smoking and cancer. Hell, the general public knew that information by the late seventies. So at least she knew about how dangerous smoking was by then. Still, she chose not to quit. She had a choice and she chose not to.

Bob: I see what you mean … I never thought about it like that.

Ted: Sad but true. No one put a gun to Carol's head and said, "You have to continue smoking or I'll kill you!" Carol made that choice all by herself. So you see, we all have choices in life that we are free to make. Destiny is not written in stone, as you say it is.

Bob: I see your point.

Ted: Also, even though Carol is a superwoman to you, she's still only a human being, and is vulnerable to the same fears and uncertainties we all face.

Bob: I guess you're right. But then is there no hope? I mean, how can we ever expect to get through the tough times, even when we *do* bring them on ourselves?

Ted: Talking with our friends and our family ultimately gets us through. We all need someone, maybe several someone's, to help us get through the tough times.

Bob: Hmm, Carol did spend a lot of time talking about the importance of having close friends, and surrounding yourself with family.

Ted: And I believe it's no accident Carol has that as a major part of her therapy, probably for just this very reason – so that you have people you can lean on during the tough times.

Bob: I guess that's true.

Ted: I'll tell you one more thing. I believe that your therapy sessions with Carol have been working for you. Over the course of the last month or so, I've seen a real change in you. Both in your attitude, and in your energy levels. There seems to be a spring in your step that wasn't there before. All of the negative self-talk has disappeared, and your outlook on life is brighter. And I'll tell you what else, you aren't such a downer to talk to anymore.

Bob: A downer? I was a downer?

Ted: You sure were. I never told you because we're such good friends, but I used to have such a headache after hanging up the phone with you. It got almost unbearable to talk with you. I was actually starting to dread our phone conversations.

Bob: Like I was an EEYORE?

Ted: Exactly! That's a very good way of putting it. You were being an EEYORE! How did you ever come up with that?

Bob: That was actually Carol's expression. She warned me about Eeyores, and told me to avoid them at all costs … now I see why.

Ted: That's why I'm so disheartened to see you abandoning your therapy because it appears to be doing you such good … at least it was. Now, it's like you're back to your old habits again, and I'm not sure how to snap you out of it.

Bob: I know, this whole thing with Carol has really thrown me for a loop. I just need some more time to figure things out, then I'll be fine. You'll see.

Ted: I sure hope so. I wish I could help you.

Bob: You have, with this phone call. Hey Ted, I need to get going, but thanks for calling to check in on me.

Ted: No problem at all, Bob. Take care, and I hope you figure things out. I'll be rooting for you!

Bob: Thanks, Ted.

———⊚———

Bob hangs up the phone. Maybe he does need Carol's help.

Carol told me to call her if I needed anything. I would also like to check on her to see how she's doing, he tells himself.

Bob decides to call Carol at home, but gets no answer. After repeated attempts, he calls Carol's office to ask the receptionist where Carol is. Bob learns that Carol has been admitted to the hospital for more testing. He decides to visit her in the hospital the next day.

CHAPTER 9

⌢

Bob Visits Carol

Bob is standing outside the front entrance to the hospital. He is hesitating. He wants to see how Carol is. However, and though he hates to admit it, he's mostly there for himself. He feels awful that he's thinking mainly of himself at a time when Carol is facing mortality.

Meekly, he slips into the hospital, tells the front desk he's there to visit his friend Carol, and asks what room she's in. It's visiting hours, so he's allowed in. Security gives him directions to Carol's room, and Bob makes his way there. He quietly knocks, then slowly enters the room when she tells him to come in.

———————⊚———————

Carol: Hello, who is it?

Bob: Uh … Hi … H … Hello Carol, it's your patient … Bob.

Carol: Oh! Hello, Bob. I wasn't expecting any visitors this morning. What a nice surprise!

Bob: I called your house yesterday, but you weren't home. I called your office, and the receptionist told me that you were in the hospital for some additional testing. I hope they didn't find that your cancer is more serious than they originally thought.

Carol: No, nothing more serious than I told you the last time we spoke. Actually, the doctors wanted to do some more tests to verify that surgery is an option for me.

Bob: That's a relief. What kind of tests are they doing, and why did you have to be admitted?

Carol: Well, the doctors know that I have a cancerous tumor in my lungs, and they have a general idea of where it is located, but they want to know its exact location so they can determine if it is operable. X-rays are not accurate enough for that purpose, so they ordered a CT scan – commonly called a "CAT Scan" – which is more precise. They also want to do some exploratory surgery. They usually do this on an outpatient basis, but because of my age, the doctors want me to stay in the hospital for a couple of days so they can keep an eye on me.

Bob: Glad it's nothing more serious than that, and that you get to go home in a day or two. I hate hospitals.

Carol: Me too. Full of sick people.

Bob: So how've you been doing since we spoke last?

Carol: I've been extremely tired. Finding out that I have lung cancer has really knocked the wind out of my sails.

Bob: I can't even imagine.

Carol: Neither could I. Throughout the years, I always knew about the risks of smoking – well, since the mid-sixties I knew – but I kept on smoking anyway. I know this is going to sound strange to you, but I never thought I would get hit by lung cancer. It just never entered my mind.

Bob: I think I understand you.

Carol: Anyway, this whole thing has been a big reminder for me; a nasty reminder actually.

Bob: What has it reminded you of?

Carol: It has reminded me that I am old, that I am not as strong as I used to be, that I am mortal, that I am not invincible. It has reminded me of how close I am to death, of how much I hate being sick, of how much I hate being tested – getting poked and prodded like a laboratory animal – and of how unpleasant hospitals are.

Bob: I'm sorry to hear that Carol, I wish there was something more I could do.

Carol: Oh, don't mind me. I'm just complaining. I guess I just needed a shoulder to cry on.

Bob: Believe me, I understand.

Carol: So how have you been? How is everything going with your daily exercises? I am eager to hear if they are making a difference for you?

Bob: I wasn't going to tell you, but they haven't been going too well lately. I've been slacking off this last week, in fact.

Carol: I knew something was going on with you by the way you entered my room; your demeanor, your posture, even your tone of voice. I could tell that something was off.

Bob: Is it that obvious?

Carol: To me it is, but only because I know what to look for. Also, I was kind of curious to see how you were doing, so I was paying extra close attention to your demeanor.

Bob: Oh, I see.

Carol: So tell me a little bit about what has been going on with you?

Bob: Well, I wasn't always feeling this way. At first, I admit I did struggle, way back at the start of our therapy sessions, I mean.

Everything seemed so hopeless. But then you forced me to complete those lists during our sessions, and followed up each week to make sure I was actually doing the exercises. As the weeks progressed, the daily exercises became easier and easier. In fact, they became part of my routine. Believe it or not, I eventually came to look forward to them. My spirits began to rise, I was in a better state of mind, and I actually started to feel physically healthier. I even made a doctor's appointment for an annual physical.

Carol: Sounds like you were on a good track. Then what happened?

Bob: You got ill. I know that sounds awful, and I don't mean to say that you were the cause of my backsliding. But, since I found out you were ill, I just haven't felt like doing much of anything really.

Carol: Tell me a little bit about how you felt once you found out I was ill.

Bob: I felt bad for you. Then I felt a rush of emotions, all at once – anger, sadness, confusion, frustration, hopelessness. Suddenly, I felt that I was not in control anymore; that is, if I ever really was in control. I started to feel anxious. Then I started to feel nervous. That quickly turned into despair, which then turned into depression and fear.

Carol: All very strong negative emotions. What was the first thing you did right after you found out I was sick?

Bob: I went to the bar.

Carol: I see. Why did you decide to go to the bar?

Bob: I don't know; I felt my anxiety welling up. All of a sudden, I felt trapped, like a caged lion. I felt I had to get out of the house and go somewhere.

Carol: And why did you choose the bar?

Bob: Because I feel comfortable there. Because it relaxes me. Because I enjoy the atmosphere. The TV is on at the bar, and that helps me pass the time. Hell, after a few drinks, I usually wind up talking with the person next to me. That helps me forget.

Carol: And what are you trying to forget?

Bob: How hopeless it all is. Let's face it, we don't have any choices in life. Take you. You didn't choose to get sick. You couldn't control that. Your sickness was pre-determined. In spite of everything that you've done to help yourself, and to help others try and be happy, it still didn't prevent this, and it certainly won't prevent death. So what's the point?

Carol: Tell me what you did the night after we spoke last; the night after you first went to the bar.

Bob: I went to the bar again.

Carol: And the next night?

Bob: I stayed home the next night; I didn't feel like going out. I ordered pizza, opened a bottle of wine, and watched some movies. In case you were wondering, I did that the next night, and the next night, and the night after that. Pretty soon, the whole week had passed.

Carol: Sounds like you have slipped back into your old routines. So tell me, what do you think caused you to slip?

Bob: I felt bad that you got sick, I guess.

Carol: Bullshit!

Bob: What?

Carol: You heard me. Now tell me why you really went to the bar that night?

Bob: I was feeling out of control, and that's what caused that rush of negative emotions. I guess you getting sick was only the catalyst, or maybe it was just an excuse, I don't know. But you *did* get sick, and you couldn't control that. You didn't choose to get sick, so maybe my fear that we have no control, no choice in life, is real. Sorry to say it, but you're living proof of that.

Carol: Now wait a minute. While it is true that we are all mortal, and that death is ultimately unavoidable, we do have control over how we live our lives while we are on this Earth. We do have control over the choices that we make.

Bob: You sure about that?

Carol: Absolutely, and I can prove it to you. I am in the medical profession, and since the mid-sixties, I knew that smoking was hazardous to my health. When the Surgeon General issued his warning publicly that cigarette smoking causes cancer, I had almost irrefutable proof that I would get cancer if I continued smoking, or at least there was a good possibility of that. Despite this, I kept right on smoking throughout all of those years. I could have quit, but I convinced myself I had become addicted, and that I couldn't quit.

I told myself that I had no choice in the matter, just as you are telling me you have no choice with the things you do. Once I was diagnosed with cancer, I realized that I had been lying to myself all those years; I realized that I did have a choice. No matter how difficult it was, I could have chosen to quit smoking. Thousands of people have quit, so I had proof that it was possible. Still, I chose to smoke. So in a way, I chose to get lung cancer. In the end, it was nobody's fault but mine.

Bob: I'm stunned! I didn't expect to hear you say you *chose* to get cancer!

Carol: I know. It's hard even for me to accept. But in a way, that's *exactly* what I did.

Now I want you to pay attention to what I say next. The reason I am telling you this is that I want you to realize we all have control over what happens to us in life, every one of us. We all have a choice. What's more, *you* have a choice. Every day, you decide what to do. Every night, you decide what to do. Tonight, you could go to the bar again, or you could stay home. You could order pizza and have wine with it, or you could have something healthier with a sparkling water. You could get up tomorrow morning and do the exercises I taught you, or not.

Bob: I see your point.

Carol: It's all about choice. It's all about *your* choice. You have a choice of what to do next. It's up to you.

Bob: Looks like I have some thinking to do this evening.

Carol: I think you do. Visiting hours are almost up. I think you had better go before the nurse comes in to kick you out. Anyway, I'm getting a bit tired, and I need to rest now.

Bob: Okay, I'll get out of your hair. Carol, thank you. I needed that.

Carol: No problem at all, Bob. I'm here anytime you need me.

Bob: At home hopefully, and not in the hospital.

Carol: I'll be home tomorrow. You can call me there if you need me.

Bob: Thanks again Carol. Get some rest, and I hope you feel better.

Carol: Thanks for coming to see me Bob. Have a good evening, and take care of yourself.

Bob: I will, Carol, goodnight.

———— ◉ ————

As Bob steps outside, a few thoughts occur to him. First, he is grateful to Carol for helping him when he needed it. Second, without even realizing it, he just had his follow-up session with Carol. Third, he begins to realize how amazing it was that Carol actually helped him, even while facing her own mortality. In fact, Carol had every right NOT to help him, and to think only of herself. Yet, she helped him anyway; regardless of her own situation.

This makes Bob realize how wonderful Carol is, and how unfair it is for her life to end this way. He starts to wonder if there is a choice in the matter.

He then realizes *he* has a choice to make for himself. He can take the new skills he has learned over the past few months and go forward in strength, or he can shrink back to the world he came from – the one he has currently lapsed back into – and die.

Bob gets in his car and heads home to ponder his choice.

TO BE CONTINUED …

ENDNOTES

⌒

Chapter 2

1. Conversano, Ciro et al. "Optimism and its impact on mental and physical well-being." Clinical practice and epidemiology in mental health : CP & EMH vol. 6 25-9. 14 May. 2010, doi:10.2174/1745017901006010025

2. Avvenuti, Giulia et al. "Optimism's Explicative Role for Chronic Diseases." Frontiers in psychology

3. "Positive Emotions and Your Health." National Institutes of Health, U.S. Department of Health and Human Services, 1 Nov. 2018, newsinhealth.nih.gov/2015/08/positive-emotions-your-health.

Chapter 3

4. Staff, Familydoctor.org Editorial. "Mind/Body Connection: How Emotions Affect Health." Familydoctor.org, 22 July 2019, familydoctor.org/mindbody-connection-how-your-emotions-affect-your-health/.

5. Rokade, P. B. "[PDF] Release of Endomorphin Hormone and Its Effects on Our Body and Moods: A Review: Semantic Scholar." [PDF] Release of Endomorphin Hormone and Its Effects on Our Body and Moods: A Review | Semantic Scholar, 1 Jan. 1970, www.semanticscholar.org/paper/Release-of-Endomorphin-Hormone-and-Its-Effects-on-A-Rokade/d9d6a77f113bb866ea1588ed-f646a60e25ca1755.

6. "Runners' High Demonstrated: Brain Imaging Shows Release Of Endorphins In Brain." ScienceDaily, ScienceDaily, 6 Mar. 2008, www.sciencedaily.com/releases/2008/03/080303101110.htm.

7. Salleh, Mohd Razali. "Life event, stress and illness." The Malaysian journal of medical sciences : MJMS vol. 15,4 (2008): 9-18.

8. Nummenmaa, Lauri et al. "Bodily maps of emotions." Proceedings of the National Academy of Sciences of the United States of America vol. 111,2 (2014): 646-51. doi:10.1073/pnas.1321664111

9. Eeyore is a character in the Winnie the Pooh books by A.A. Milne, first published in 1926.

10. "The Law of Compensation: Emerson Essays." Ralph Waldo Emerson, 1841, emersoncentral.com/texts/essays-first-series/compensation/.

11. Ibid.

12. Smith, Lee et al. "Sexual Activity is Associated with Greater Enjoyment of Life in Older Adults." Sexual medicine vol. 7,1 (2019): 11-18. doi:10.1016/j.esxm.2018.11.001

13. Ibid.

14. Gawain, Shakti, and Marci Shimoff. *Creative Visualization: Use the Power of Your Imagination to Create What You Want in Your Life.* New World Library, 2016.

Chapter 4

15. "Alcohol's Effects on the Body." *National Institute on Alcohol Abuse and Alcoholism*, U.S. Department of Health and Human Services, 6 June 2019, www.niaaa.nih.gov/alcohols-effects-body.

16. "Karpman Drama Triangle." Wikipedia, Wikimedia Foundation, 25 Mar. 2020, en.wikipedia.org/wiki/Karpman_drama_triangle.

17. Karpman, Stephen B. *A Game Free Life: the Definitive Book on the Drama Triangle and the Compassion Triangle by the Originator and Author.* Drama Triangle Productions, 2014.

18. Ibid Note 10.

Chapter 5

19. Staff, Mayo Clinic. "How to Stop Negative Self-Talk." *Mayo Clinic*, Mayo Foundation for Medical Education and Research, 18 Feb. 2017, www.mayoclinic.org/healthy-lifestyle/stress-management/in-depth/positive-thinking/art-20043950.

20. Rippon, Isla. "Feeling Old vs Being Old." *JAMA Internal Medicine*, American Medical Association, 1 Feb. 2015, jamanetwork.com/journals/jamainternalmedicine/fullarticle/2020288.

21. Lee, Lewina O., et al. "Optimism Is Associated with Exceptional Longevity in 2 Epidemiologic Cohorts of Men and Women." PNAS, National Academy of Sciences, 10 Sept. 2019, www.pnas.org/content/116/37/18357.

22. Sirois, F. M. (2015). Is procrastination a vulnerability factor for hypertension and cardiovascular disease? Testing an extension of the procrastination–health model. *Journal of Behavioral Medicine*, 1-12. doi: 10.1007/s10865-015-9629-2

23. Park, Denise C et al. "The impact of sustained engagement on cognitive function in older adults: the Synapse Project." *Psychological science* vol. 25,1 (2014): 103-12. doi:10.1177/0956797613499592

24. University Of Toronto. "Old Brains Can Learn New Tricks: Study Shows Older People Use Different Areas Of The Brain To Perform Same 'Thinking Task' As Young." ScienceDaily. ScienceDaily, 25 October 1999. <www.sciencedaily.com/releases/1999/10/991021094811.htm>.

25. McGillivray, Shannon et al. "Thirst for knowledge: The effects of curiosity and interest on memory in younger and older adults." *Psychology and aging* vol. 30,4 (2015): 835-41. doi:10.1037/a0039801

26. Gómez-Pinilla, Fernando. "Brain foods: the effects of nutrients on brain function." *Nature reviews. Neuroscience* vol. 9,7 (2008): 568-78. doi:10.1038/nrn2421

Chapter 6

27. Wells, Brent. "Chiropractic From the Feet Up: How Your Feet Impact Your Whole Body." *Better Health Chiropractic*, 19 Aug. 2019, betterhealthalaska.com/chiropractic-from-the-feet-up-how-your-feet-impact-your-whole-body/.

28. Embong, Nurul Haswani et al. "Revisiting reflexology: Concept, evidence, current practice, and practitioner training." *Journal of traditional and complementary medicine* vol. 5,4 197-206. 28 Sep. 2015, doi:10.1016/j.jtcme.2015.08.008

29. Katon, Wayne J. "Epidemiology and treatment of depression in patients with chronic medical illness." *Dialogues in clinical neuroscience* vol. 13,1 (2011): 7-23.

30. Levine, Hallie. "When Do You Need to See a Geriatric Specialist?" *AARP*, 11 Feb. 2019, www.aarp.org/health/conditions-treatments/info-2019/geriatrics-specialist.html.

31. "Aging Changes in Skin: MedlinePlus Medical Encyclopedia." *MedlinePlus*, U.S. National Library of Medicine, Apr. 2020, medlineplus.gov/ency/article/004014.htm.

32. Gouin, Jean-Philippe, and Janice K Kiecolt-Glaser. "The Impact of Psychological Stress on Wound Healing: Methods and Mechanisms." Immunology and Allergy Clinics of North America, U.S. National Library of Medicine, Feb. 2011, www.ncbi.nlm.nih.gov/pmc/articles/PMC3052954/.

33. Emery, Charles F, et al. "Exercise Accelerates Wound Healing among Healthy Older Adults: a Preliminary Investigation." *The Journals of Gerontology. Series A, Biological Sciences and Medical Sciences*, U.S. National Library of Medicine, Nov. 2005, www.ncbi.nlm.nih.gov/pubmed/16339330.

34. Lin, Frank R, and Marilyn Albert. "Hearing loss and dementia - who is listening?." *Aging & mental health* vol. 18,6 (2014): 671-3. doi:10.1080/13607863.2014.915924

35. "Vision Health & Age| Risk." *Centers for Disease Control and Prevention*, Centers for Disease Control and Prevention, 28 Sept. 2009, www.cdc.gov/vision-health/risk/age.htm.

36. Lilleston, Randy. "STD Rates Continue to Rise for Older Adults." *AARP*, 28 Sept. 2017, www.aarp.org/health/conditions-treatments/info-2017/std-exposure-rises-older-adults-fd.html.

APPENDIX A

Spirit Exercises

The following are a set of exercises designed to help you elevate your spirits and put you into a positive emotional state, which is one of the keys to unlocking the doors to happiness, health, and fulfillment. Please complete the exercises below as best as you can.

Be thankful for what you have

In the table below, list out at least 10 things that you are thankful for. If you need more space, you can use the blank *Notes* pages at the end of the book.

1) _____

2) _____

3) _____

4) _____

5) _____

6) _____

7) _____

8) _____

9) _____

10) _____

11) _____

12) _____

13) _____

14) _____

15) _____

Surround yourself with family

In the table below, make a list of your family members. This list can include either blood relatives, adopted family, or both. Next to the name of each family member, write the current state of your relationship with them. For example, is your relationship with them good, or is it strained? How close do you currently feel to them, very close or very distant? How do you feel emotionally when you think of them? Do you feel happy, or angry, or sad?

If you are not on good terms with a particular family member, it will also help to write down what caused the relationship to become strained. This will give you a perspective that might prove helpful when you begin to repair the relationship.

If you need more space, you can use the blank *Notes* pages at the end of the book.

Have close friends

Review the list of family members you compiled as part of the second technique – **Surround yourself with family**, and add the names of your close friends. For each person on your updated list, mark whether they are an Eeyore. If you need more space, you can use the blank *Notes* pages at the end of the book.

Be happy for others' good fortune

Think of something good that has happened to each person on your list of family and friends, and write that next to their name. If you need more space, you can use the blank *Notes* pages at the end of the book.

Name of Family Member or Friend	Current State of Relationship	Cause of Strained Relationship (Optional)	A Good Thing That Happened to Them	EEYORE? (Yes/No)
1)				
2)				
3)				
4)				
5)				
6)				
7)				
8)				
9)				
10)				
11)				
12)				
13)				
14)				
15)				

Look at the beauty of nature around you

In the table below, write down at least 10 things that you find beautiful in nature. If you need more space, you can use the blank *Notes* pages at the end of the book.

1) _____

2) _____

3) _____

4) _____

5) _____

6) _____

7) _____

8) _____

9) _____

10) _____

11) _____

12) _____

13) _____

14) _____

15) _____

Do something for someone else

Make a list of at least 10 things you have done for someone else. These things could either be in the recent or distant past. Next to each item, write down how that good deed made you feel, and how you were compensated for it. Remember, your compensation does not necessarily come from the person you did the good deed for, nor does it necessarily immediately follow the good deed. Compensation can come days, months, or even years afterward.

If you do not recognize how you were compensated for a specific action, just leave a blank next to it. However, for each action on your list, do write down how it made you feel. That part is important.

If you need more space, you can use the blank *Notes* pages at the end of the book.

AFTER 60

Person's Name	The Good Deed You Did for Them	How it Made You Feel	How You Were Compensated
1)			
2)			
3)			
4)			
5)			
6)			
7)			
8)			
9)			
10)			
11)			
12)			
13)			
14)			
15)			

Do the things you enjoy doing

Make a list of at least 10 things you enjoy doing. You can put anything on this list, whether you have done it yet or not. You might include only enjoyable things that you have done in the past, but you can also include things that you have not done yet, but might enjoy doing in the future.

If you want to add routine chores to your list, create two sub-categories, one called "Enjoyment" and one called "Chores." You can then add both types of activities to the same list. If you build your list this way, try to balance the activities you enjoy doing with the activities that are chores. Try to make sure you have at least a 50/50 split. A 70/30 split is better.

If you need more space, you can use the blank *Notes* pages at the end of the book.

Activity Description	Sub-Category (Enjoyment / Chores)
1)	
2)	
3)	
4)	
5)	
6)	
7)	
8)	
9)	
10)	
11)	
12)	
13)	
14)	
15)	

Find some way to release your frustrations

In the table below, make a list of 10 physical activities you can engage in when you become frustrated. They can be any safe activity that is physical. The key is to identify activities you can do as soon as you become frustrated. If you need more space, you can use the blank *Notes* pages at the end of the book.

1) _____

2) _____

3) _____

4) _____

5) _____

6) _____

7) _____

8) _____

9) _____

10) _____

11) _____

12) _____

13) _____

14) _____

15) _____

APPENDIX B

⌐

Mind Exercises

The following are a set of exercises designed to help put you into a positive mental state, which is one of the keys to unlocking the doors to happiness, health, and fulfillment. Please complete the exercises below as best as you can.

Live in the present

Write down how your life has been improved by either modern conveniences, technology, or medical advances. First list each item, then briefly write about how it has improved your life. You do not need to come up with an item for each category, the point of the exercise is to think about how things in the world today make your life better. If you need more space, you can use the blank *Notes* pages at the end of the book.

Item Description	Category (Modern Conveniences/ Technology/ Medical Advances)	How it has Improved Your Life
1)		
2)		
3)		
4)		
5)		
6)		
7)		
8)		
9)		
10)		
11)		
12)		
13)		
14)		
15)		

Do it now

The table below is a template that you can use as a starting point for your own personal To-Do list. Feel free to customize it according to what works best for you.

TO-DOs			
Task Description	Time Needed to Complete (In Hours)	Due Date	Done (Yes/No)
1)			
2)			
3)			
4)			
5)			
6)			
7)			
8)			
9)			
10)			
11)			
12)			
13)			
14)			
15)			

APPENDIX C

List of Techniques

The following are the lists of MIND, BODY, and SPIRIT techniques covered in the book. We have included these here for your reference.

Spirit
1) Be thankful for what you have
2) Surround yourself with family
3) Have close friends, but choose them wisely
4) Be happy for others' good fortune
5) Look at the beauty of nature around you
6) Do something for someone else
7) Do the things you enjoy doing
8) Find some way to release your frustrations

Mind
1) Keep informed
2) Keep up your physical appearance
3) Live your life regardless of your age
4) Live in the present
5) Push yourself to participate
6) Do it now
7) Keep your mind fit
8) Keep in touch with time
9) Continue to learn

Body
1) Go to a podiatrist
2) See your doctor at least once a year
3) Get your blood work done once a year
4) Have a doctor look at sores that are not healing
5) Have your ears and your eyes checked
6) Maintain good dental health
7) Keep active physically
8) Do things in moderation

ABOUT THE AUTHORS

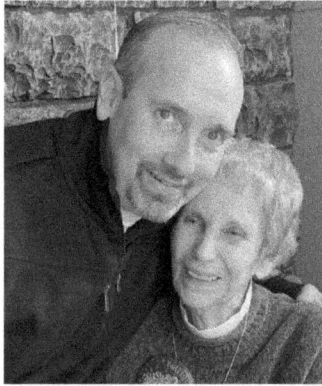

Audrey C. Ralph

Audrey C. Ralph is a retired registered nurse who spent over 25 years in the field of geriatric care, first as a nursing supervisor, then as a geriatric in-home care specialist. During her career, she helped those in her care to live happier, healthier, and more fulfilled lives. She spent her early career as a public health nurse, then worked as a nursing supervisor for the Visiting Nurses Association of New York – working in New York City and Spanish Harlem. In her later years, she gained knowledge and experience caring for older patients, first as a nursing supervisor at Rydal Park Medical Center, then as an in-home care specialist.

Audrey was born and grew up in Hamden, Connecticut. She had an older sister named Dorothy, who worked as a bank teller and secretary. Her mother was a full-time homemaker, and her father was an officer in a plumbing supply company in New Haven, Connecticut.

She trained as a registered nurse at Grace New Haven School of Nursing. She went on to get her Bachelor of Science in Nursing Education from Syracuse University, and her Master of Science in Nursing Education from Yale University.

Audrey enjoys activities such as singing in various church groups, gardening, reading, natural science, and being with family and friends. She lives in Fort Washington, Pennsylvania.

Gordon Ralph

Gordon Ralph is the Founder and CEO of Ternion Press, LLC – the company that publishes the *Life After 60*™ series.

His career has spanned more than 30 years, during which time he has served as an entrepreneur, accountant, computer systems analyst, business consultant, career coach, photographer, programmer, and author.

Gordon was born and raised in a suburb of Philadelphia, Pennsylvania. He received his Bachelor of Science in Accounting from Drexel University in Philadelphia, Pennsylvania, and earned an M.B.A. in Entrepreneurship from Babson College in Wellesley, Massachusetts.

Gordon is an avid reader and enjoys practicing and playing golf, photography, and drawing. He is married and works in Portland, Oregon.

NOTES

NOTES

NOTES

NOTES

NOTES